Sexuality healthcare: dilem

Sexuality and healthcare: a human dilemma

Edited by
Matthew V. Morrissey

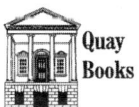
Quay Books

Quay Books Division, Mark Allen Publishing Group
Jesses Farm, Snow Hill, Dinton, Wiltshire, SP3 5HN

British Library Cataloguing-in-Publication Data
A catalogue record is available for this book

©Mark Allen Publishing 1998
ISBN 1 85642 095 7

All rights reserved. No part of this publication may be reproduced, stored in a retrieval system or transmitted in any form or by any means, electronic, mechanical, photocopying, recording or otherwise, without prior permission from the publishers.

Printed in the UK by Redwood Books, Trowbridge, Wiltshire.

Contents

List of contributors		vii
Acknowledgements		ix
Preface		xi
Introduction		xiii
Part 1: Overview and theoretical issues		1
1	Making sense of sexuality : *David T Evans*	3
2	Multiple positions: a philosophical approach to sexual health : *Robert-Gareth Hill*	39
3	Psychological perspectives on human sexuality : *Ian Rivers*	61
4	Sexuality and childbirth: towards a theory of female sexuality : *Anna Sobolewski*	75
Part 2: Meeting the needs of specific client groups		93
5	Healthcare for lesbian, gay and bisexual individuals : *Matthew V Morrissey*	95
6	Sexuality and the child : *Cherry Bennett*	115
7	The pregnant adolescent: sexually ignorant or destroyer of society's values? : *Tessa Muncey*	127
8	Health and people with learning disabilities : *Tony Gilbert*	159
9	Sexuality and mental health: challenging ignorance and prejudice *Matthew V Morrissey*	173
Part 3: Evaluating practice		187
10	Sexuality, nursing and professional practice: *Shirley Crouch*	189
11	Perspectives on sexual health promotion: *Theodore H MacDonald*	209
12	Sexuality and sexual health: towards a dynamic nursing curriculum : *Matthew Morrissey and Shirley Crouch*	225
Appendix		237

Contacts 239

Index 243

Contributors

Cherry Bennett is a Senior Lecturer at Homerton College Cambridge, School of Health Studies, Peterborough District Hospital, Thorpe Road, Peterborough, PE3 6DA. Her interests include child and adolescent development and paediatric nursing.

Shirley Crouch is a Senior Lecturer at Homerton College Cambridge, School of Health Studies, Peterborough District Hospital, Thorpe Road, Peterborough, PE3 6DA. Her interests include elderly care, ethics and professional practice. Presently studying for a PhD.

David T Evans is a Senior Lecturer in Sociology at the University of Glasgow. He has published a number of articles on sociology. His writings on sexuality include: Sexual Citizenship: The Material Construction of Sexualities (Routledge 1993).

Tony Gilbert is Head of Department: Community and Primary Health Care at Homerton College Cambridge, Fulborne Hospital Education Centre, Ida Darwin Hospital, Fulborne, Cambridge, CB1 5EE. He has published widely in the area of sociology and learning disability. He has worked in a range of services for adults and children with learning disabilities. His present research interest is in the area of how trust is constructed in professional roles.

Robert-Gareth Hill was previously a Research Associate with the Sainsbury Centre for Mental Health. He is, at present, undertaking a D.Psych in Clinical Psychology and completing a PhD. Research interests include: philosophy, manic depression, existential psychology and mental health.

Professor Theodore MacDonald is Director of Postgraduate Studies in Health at Brunel University College, London. He has held university chairs in: Education, Mathematics and Medicine in various countries and has practised as a general practitioner both in the UK and abroad. He has published over 160 research papers and 30 books. General interests include: classics, music, animals and politics.

Matthew V Morrissey is a Senior Lecturer (Mental Health) at Canterbury Christ Church College. Research interests include: mental health, human rights, Alzheimer's disease and elderly care, and sexuality and healthcare.

Tessa Muncey is Academic Director at Homerton College Cambridge, School of Health Studies, Education Centre, Addenbrookes Hospital, Cambridge, CB2 2QQ. Research interests include: women's health, psychology and teenage pregnancy. She is at present undertaking a PhD.

Ian Rivers is a Lecturer in Psychology at the University of Luton. He has published widely in the area of bullying in adolescence in relation to gay and lesbian youth, nationally and internationally. He is currently completing his PhD in this area. He is a Fellow of the International Society for Research on Aggression, and has been a guest speaker at universities in Italy, Sweden and the United States.

Anna Sobolewski is a Senior Lecturer in Women's Health at the University of Central England. She was born in California and is a qualified midwife. She completed a Masters degree in Health Psychology in 1995. Her interests include: women's health, midwifery practice and health psychology.

Acknowledgements

Many people have helped in the preparation of this text. We cannot name everyone but would like to extend our warmest thanks to:

- Nursing Students at Canterbury Christ Church College
- Professor Sue Holmes and Professor Stephen Clift
- Corrine, Barbera, Linda, Sue, Pat, and Tania in Cambridge
- David Whitworth-Judd, Caroline Fenn, Chris Biela
- James, Elizabeth and Claire Robinson, Paul Cobb, Geoff Henning
- Matthew and Mary, Kenneth and Valerie, Jennifer and Nicole
- Chantelle, Sonya, Kevin, Fiona and Paudy, Darragh and Cian
- Special thanks to Brenda Didmon and Valery Marston
- Dennis Dorman, Karen Worden and Louise Holland.

Special thanks also to families and friends for their patience and support in this creative project. Any errors or omissions are those of the respective authors and the views expressed by authors are not necessarily those of their employing organisations.

Matthew V Morrissey
Department of Nursing
Canterbury Christ Church College
November 1997

Preface

This text provides an exploration of sexuality in relation to healthcare. It combines a critical approach to theory and practice and is compiled as a textbook for healthcare professionals and those studying courses in healthcare and related subjects.

There has been a substantial development in degree and postgraduate courses in nursing and healthcare. Intrinsic to many of these is the study of human sexuality. Not only do healthcare workers need to understand issues relating to this area but, increasingly, they need knowledge and skills in practice. Furthermore, the development of a policy in many areas where sexuality is affected directly and indirectly by healthcare practices is essential. The text offers a collection of perspectives that promote the understanding of human sexuality and healthcare as a human rather than biological dilemma. Healthcare workers are frequently involved in care and need to feel comfortable with the final frontier — sexuality.

Introduction

Matthew V. Morrissey

Historically the topic of sex and sexuality has been cloaked in mystery and taboo. These areas of our lives have been, and to some extent still are, interpreted and ruled primarily by religion, morality and the law. Many types of discourse, both informal and academic, exist on the topic and there is no shortage of literature. However, there is a real need to examine issues connected with sexuality for health professionals. To some extent what guides health professionals is the recognition of the global and international context and diversity of healthcare. If healthcare and health promotion are to be effective in improving sexual health there is a need to affirm sexuality not pathologise it.

Research has shown that nurses are reluctant to discuss sexuality issues with clients. Much of this reluctance is the result of embarrassment, lack of healthcare policies in practice and, more importantly, a lack of confidence and skill in dealing with such personal issues (Waterhouse, 1996; Kantz *et al*, 1990). When healthcare professionals and nurses are given the opportunity to explore sexuality issues, a more positive approach is adopted (Frazer, 1982; Matocha and Waterhouse, 1993). There is, however, a need to examine aspects of the curriculum surrounding education in sexual health and sexuality for health professionals. The curricula need to be updated to include content which has not previously been included. There is a need to focus on issues relating to attitudes and skills not just knowledge. Furthermore, methods of evaluating clinical practice in relation to sexual health should be established. If health professionals are to provide individual care it is important to treat the person in a holistic way. Clearly this means integrating sex and sexuality as part of healthcare, but sadly, many health professionals feel inadequately prepared.

Recent publications have documented the lack of appropriate preparation of many healthcare workers, including nurses, in dealing with issues related to sex and sexuality (Rose, 1994; Grigg, 1997). Education is essential for healthcare workers who often feel unprepared for this aspect of their role (Waterhouse, 1996; Purdie, 1996). However, education for health professionals needs to focus more on debate and discussion concerning methods of working and education (Morrissey *et al*, in press).

Exploring issues in relation to sexuality is important in healthcare where professionals, such as nurses, often work with clients in a direct, close and personal way. However, education is particularly important for young people after surgery in relation to disability, mental health and pregnancy (Albarran and Bridger, 1997; Knapp, 1997; O'Toole, 1996; Parrillo et al, 1997; Stephany, 1992; Waxman, 1996). Medicine historically dissects and depersonalises subjects like sexuality into a biological rather than social phenomenon. It is important to realise that human sexuality is dynamic and a human, rather than a simply biological, fact.

This book is divided into three sections: dealing with theoretical issues, meeting the needs of specific client groups and evaluating health promotion practice with respect to sexuality in the context of healthcare. In each section contributors explore issues of concern to health professionals when considering their role in addressing sexuality in the context of healthcare.

In *Section 1* theoretical issues are examined in relation to sociology, philosophy, psychology and female sexuality. The first chapter in this section examines sexuality from a sociological perspective and includes definitions and representations of sexuality in society and the media; *Chapter 2* examines the contribution that philosophy can make to our understanding of human sexuality. This chapter offers a critical analysis of definitions and concepts surrounding sexual health. *Chapter 3* reviews sexuality from a psychological perspective, focusing on an examination of the ways in which sexuality has been studied, the normality/abnormality debate within psychology and redefining normality in terms of cultural diversity. *Chapter 4* critically examines sexuality and childbirth; included here is a review of research and theory in relation to female sexuality, historical and psychological perspectives, the biological perspective, the cultural perspective, lesbian mothers and suggestions on rethinking definitions of female sexuality.

Section 2 examines ways of meeting the sexual health needs of specific client groups including gay, lesbian and bisexual clients, children, teenagers, people with learning disabilities and mental health. *Chapter 5* discusses the health-care needs of lesbian, gay and bisexual clients. Areas covered include: homosexuality and society, public opinion and public policy, a brief history of homosexuality and healthcare, law, religion and homosexuality, and attitudes of health professionals to clients who are lesbian, gay or bisexual.

Chapter 6 investigates issues surrounding sexuality and the child. In this chapter, the author outlines how children learn about sexuality, child development in relation to self-image, sexuality and childcare and an examination of the way forward. *Chapter 7* extends this further by examining teenage pregnancy in a wider and more challenging perspective in relation to the debate on childhood sexuality. The chapter covers the health carer's perspective, health risks, childhood sexuality, and the myth of childhood innocence and broken images.

Sexual health in relation to people with learning disabilities is discussed in *Chapter 8*. First the author examines the problem of sexuality in the biological and social context and then goes on to discuss issues connected with gender and sexuality, sexuality, pleasure and identity. *Chapter 9* considers sexuality in relation to mental health suggesting that people with mental health problems are also marginalised in a similar way to those with a learning disability. It is suggested that, if progress is to be made, sexuality must be seen as part of human relationships and not as part of a mental illness. Furthermore, it is suggested that the development of policies in mental health settings must protect clients from abuse, rape and violence. Clients need to be empowered in the area of sexuality and informed about drugs, situations which could compromise their sexuality and personal safety. Research in the area of mental health and sexuality is reviewed and recommendations made for better and more informed practice.

The final section of this book suggests ways of evaluating practice. In *Chapter 10* nursing, sexuality and professional practice are examined in relation to the following areas: sexuality towards a definition, sexuality and the well-being of the individual, beliefs, values and attitudes, patients rights, meeting sexuality needs, and education and training. *Chapter 11* examines ways of evaluating sexual health promotion. It includes a review in relation to HIV/AIDS, outlining the issues to be discussed, empowerment and preventative strategies, social and psychological constraints, medicalisation verses health promotion, trust, intimacy and personal autonomy, perception of risk, the problems of assessment and critique of evaluation.

Chapter 12 summarises the issues raised in the previous chapters and suggests ways of providing a more dynamic curriculum to teach those working in healthcare. In particular, it is suggested that many issues need to be included in relation to sexuality in the curriculum. Issues, such as childhood sexuality, healthcare for lesbian, gay and bisexual clients, female sexuality and childbirth, learning disability and mental health have previously been excluded resulting in a narrow focus on human sexuality. It is hoped that such a discussion will provide ideas and a basic foundation for those working in healthcare practice and education.

This text aims to:
- explore the theoretical aspects and meanings of sexuality in society generally and in healthcare practice specifically

- examine issues relating to meeting the needs of specific client groups in healthcare
- evaluate current health promotion practices and education with respect to sexuality in the context of healthcare
- outline a suitable curriculum model for the education and training of healthcare professionals in sexuality.

References

Albarran JW, Bridger S (1997) Problems with providing education on resuming sexual activity after myocardial infarction: developing written information for patients. *Inten Crit Care Nurs* **13**(1): 2–11

Frazer J (1982) Impact of a human sexuality workshop on the sexual attitudes and knowledge of nursing students. *J Nurs Educ* **21**(3): 6–13

Grigg E (1997) Guidelines for teaching about sexuality. *Nurse Educ Today* **17**(1): 62–6

Kantz DD, Dickey CA, Stevens MN (1990) Using research to identify why nurses do not meet established sexuality nursing care standards. *J Nurs Qual Ass* **4**(3): 69–78

Knapp J (1997) Sexual function as a quality of life issue: the impact of breast cancer treatment. *Gynecolog Oncol Nurs* **7**(1): 37–40

Matocha LK, Waterhouse JK (1993) Current nursing practice related to sexuality. *Res Nurs Health* **16**: 371–8

Morrissey M, Rivers I (1998) Applying the Mims-Swenson Sexual Health Model to nurse education: A focus on sexuality and healthcare. *Nurse Educ Today* **18**: 488–95

O'Toole CJ (1996) Disabled lesbians: challenging monocultural constructs *Sexual Disabil* **14**(3): 221–36.

Parillo AV, Felts WM, Mikow-Porto V (1997) Early initiation of sexual intercourse and its co-occurence with other health risk-behaviours in high school students: the 1993 North Carolina Youth Risk Behaviour Survey. *J Health Educ* **28**(2): 85–96

Purdie H (1996) Management of sexuality in a mental health setting. *Nurs Stand* **11**(12): 47–50

Rose L (1994) Homophobia among doctors. *Br Med J* **308**: 586–7

Stephany TM (1992) Promoting mental health: lesbian nurse support groups. *J Psychosoc Nurs* **30**(2): 35–8

Waterhouse J (1996) Nursing practice related to sexuality: a review and recommendations. *Nurs Times Res* 1(6): 412–8

Waxman BF (1996) Commentary on sexual and reproductive health. *Sexual Disabil* **14**(3): 221–36

Part 1
Overview and theoretical issues

1
Making sense of sexuality

David T Evans

'Safer sex is a culturally differentiated process . . . Sex is a social activity, an interaction subject to negotiation' (Pollak, 1994).

The 'sexual fix'

Society is preoccupied by sexuality, taking it very seriously indeed, but rarely attempting to consider it rationally. The rapid sexualisation of modern societies cannot be doubted. It has been variously described as becoming hooked on the 'sexual fix' (Heath 1982), 'worshipping at the altar of sex religion' (Greer 1984), and especially since 'the rutting revolution' of the 'permissive 60s' (Amis 1985). Sexuality has become 'the medium through which people . . . define their personalities', establish their identities, 'become conscious of themselves' (Foucault 1981). Sexual 'knowledge' is delivered in all manner of forms, from the bible, medical texts and sex education in schools, comics, fashion-spreads, TV soap operas, jokes, advertisements, pop songs and feature films. Bodies' dimensions are measured, their inadequacies hopefully rectified by exercise, diet or plastic surgery. Sexual dysfunctions such as impotence are diagnosed and treated. 'Victims' of any sexual shortcoming or offence are counselled into being 'survivors'. Sexual 'types' are meticulously catalogued. 'Perfect' sex acts are choreographed and trained for. In all these respects we are driven to achieve perfect fulfilment and happiness through the realisation of our personal 'innermost', 'unique', sexual souls, and to help us further in this quest, we consult all manner of 'experts': doctors, teachers, psychiatrists, priests, best friends, agony aunts, astrology charts and, vicariously, chat show hosts, such as, Oprah, Montel, Ricki, Vanessa and Esther.

Furthermore, sexuality, or to be more accurate sexual*ties* for there are many forms in modern societies, have become associated with everything requiring explanation no matter how minor or apparently non-sexual. Sexual images sell cars, chocolate bars, kitchens, holidays, perfumes, aftershaves, jeans, Coke and Pepsi. As a result, sexuality in a conventional sense tends to evaporate, for it is inextricably tied up with all aspects of our lives in what has been called our contemporary culture of 'bio-power' (Foucault 1981). If this sounds like a wonder detergent then it is apt, for 'bio-power' refers to our obsessions with all aspects of our appearance: bodily health and maintenance, its cosmetic presentation in behaviour and consumer products, such as designer clothes etc, of which sexuality, in the narrow, conventional sense, forms the core. All are displayed, like one's 'whiter than whites', to a critically appraising world. Thus 'bio-power' is the 'grouping together in an artificial unity . . . (of) anatomical elements, biological functions, conducts, sensations and pleasures, and (makes) use of this fictitious unity as a causal principle, an omnipresent meaning, a secret to be discovered everywhere' (Foucault, 1981). But this is where society encounters the ambiguity of this 'bio-power' culture. We may be obsessed by matters sexual in the narrow sense of 'who does what to whom, when, where and how', but seldom are we conscious of the implicit sexual 'knowledge' of the messages and images with which we are bombarded on a daily mundane basis.

From these brief examples, it should be clear that sex is not simply a biological phenomenon. In our culture of 'bio-power', we are led to believe that it is a 'mysterious' force of nature, not the product of our social environment. We believe patterns of sexual behaviour and sexual values are governed by universal biological drives. Simultaneously, we are also driven to uncover the innermost natural 'secrets' of, what we believe to be, our own 'unique' sexual beings. In effect, our culture of 'bio-power' consists of a long-running hoax. We are deceived into explaining sexuality through nature, yet all the time 'sexualities' are constructed and moulded by dynamic social and cultural influences. Our familiar patterns of sexual behaviour norms, conventions and obsessions are not found in all human populations. Nor have they been constant features of our own history. Rather, they are culturally and historically specific, which is why Foucault describes 'bio-power' as an 'artificial' and a 'fictitious unity'. We sexual and sex-obsessed beings are the product of our time and place, not our genes, and our sexualities are not merely the products of our sex-obsessed culture, but of the specific social, political and economic conditions within which we live. As we shall see, we are not merely bombarded by sexual messages and images, we find ourselves increasingly consumers of sexual and sexualised commodities in a leisure economy, and our sexual identities are associated with considerable political and moral monitoring by the state through the differential citizenship rights and responsibilities formally associated with them.

It is not surprising that any attempt to make sense of the social construction of sexualities in our society, normally commences by focusing on cultural messages and images, especially those transmitted through the mass media. Daily media coverage of specific sexual issues is considerable, as a brief listing of some currently of interest reminds us:

- rising divorce rates
- rape trial procedures
- 'date-rape'
- developments in IV-fertilisation
- cloning and its legal controls
- the marketing of drugs, such as Viagra, to 'cure' impotence
- sexual discrimination in the armed forces
- 'safe sex'
- all aspects of AIDS
- sex education in schools
- the problematic rehabilitation of 'paedophiles in the community'
- the operations of the Child Support Agency etc.

More insidious however, because seemingly unimportant, is the sexual 'knowledge' found in informal media discourses such as advertising images, gossip columns, texts of pop songs, plots of films, themes and gags of comedy and plot-lines of 'soaps'. In some instances we are conscious of the sexual components, as with Benetton's use of a 'real' AIDS 'victim' to sell its sweaters and Peugeot's use of a suggested all-male kiss to sell their 306 model ('Search for the hero inside yourself' sang the accompanying Heather Small voice-over). We are unlikely to consciously recognise the sexual elements in Safeway's use of 'cute' children mimicking adults to sell their domestic produce: the middle-class housewife's use of Ariel or the late Princess Di's, designer clad, obsessive gym workouts to counter rumoured upper thigh cellulite. But the sexual is present in all of these images and messages which idealise certain sexual ways of looking and living, thereby exerting 'biopower'.

On television, sexual 'knowledge' mostly comes in trivial repetitive, commonplace forms — Tony Blair tells 'mother-in-law' jokes on the Des O'Connor Show, yet such 'knowledge', as with the formal instruction of medical, religious, legal and other texts, and the language through which it is communicated, is suffused with power, hence 'bio-power'. It influences us in terms of the words we use, the opinions we form and the behaviour we enact, to believe that we are first and foremost sexually, biologically driven and not the product of these very same social forces.

Our everyday language is full of sexual innuendo, slang, and joking which signify the seriousness with which we treat sexual matters, but which also demonstrates that these cannot be discussed openly, without embarrassment. Sex is of central importance, but viewed as a 'secret'. Thus we use short-hand stereotypes to classify the 'good' and the 'bad', the 'normal' and the 'perverse', 'right' and 'wrong', implying that the 'good', 'normal' and 'right' are naturally so. The power implications are nowhere more evident than in the familiar slang, which from our earliest peer group play, keeps males and females under informal social and sexual control: 'queer', 'poof', 'slut', 'tart' and 'whore' (Lees, 1993: Mac an Ghaill, 1994). These labels are reputational straightjackets which warn us, even before we fully know what they mean, to monitor our behaviours in front of others, for fear of 'name-calling' sanctions, ridicule or physical attack. Indeed, our learning of these terms in our most formative years establishes our lifelong obsession with sex as something dark, threatening and secretive. Such terms, even when used by four- or five-year-olds, are hardly power-neutral, nor are their alternatives, 'gay' and 'dyke'. In our culture, in fact in any culture, even technical terms carry judgmental implications; the '. . . apparently neutral description of men as either heterosexual or homosexual since the nineteenth century conceals the intricate play of power, of domination and subordination which minoritises the homosexual experience and consolidates male power in a new effective pattern' (Woodhead 1995).

In summary, we believe that sexuality is the most natural and private part of our beings and yet we are constantly thinking about it, talking about it, expressing opinions about it. Sex is not something that just *is*, which we then describe and judge, it is something which is socially and culturally shaped by even the most mundane 'knowledge' we learn and use. As references to 'bio-power' suggest, our obsession with sexuality is as much with the cosmetic promise of the sexual — the presentation of the body as fit and 'healthy', a well-groomed and dressed sexual machine — as it is with the actual mechanics of sex. We aspire to the purchase of expensive designer-labelled clothes to set off an all-year 'healthy' tan and flashing, capped, white teeth. Such is the wrapping which implicitly promises the discovery of a 'secret' gift of our individual sexual identities, and it does not come cheap. Making sense of sexuality requires an exploration of the complex and dynamic ways in which sexualities are socially and politically constructed. This is hidden behind the fundamental cultural belief that they are simply the result of universal natural laws. Indeed, as we shall see, the blind certainty of this belief is a crucial element in their social construction.

Common-sense

As with all other aspects of behaviour, human sexualities can only be explained by addressing their social organisation and cultural meanings in particular societies at specific stages in their historical development. Cross-culturally, sexual conventions vary across the entire spectrum of acts, relationships and institutions. Male same-sex acts can be fundamental components of sexual norms, whether as aspects of adolescent rites of passage or of respected adult roles and relationships (Mead, 1935). Children, regarded in our own culture as sexual innocents, may in others be socialised into sexual acts of various kinds from early ages (Evans, 1993), and marital and family institutions take numerous forms from serial or simultaneous polygamy and polyandry, to monogamy (Harris, 1970).

In all such instances, prevailing cultural conventions are perceived as naturally right and 'God-given', sustained by common-sense explanations, informally inducing broad behavioural conformity and justifying sanctions for those who deviate. For readers tempted to draw ethnocentric conclusions from such comparisons with what they might perceive as less developed cultures, it should be pointed out that if, as geneticists claim, there is no evidence of racially differentiated biologies, universal human sexual 'truths' would have to be apparent in all populations, whatever their level and form of development, and this is simply not the case.

In addition, histories of single cultures reveal often dramatic changes in approved sexual behaviours over relatively short periods. Recent British history manifests, as do all societies with capital growth economies, a constant restructuring and redefinition of sexual conventions and norms. Childhood sexual innocence, for example, is very much a product of nineteenth century social and legal reforms, as are the gendered and sexual roles of women and men within and outside the nuclear family. Yet boys of 12 years of age are now legally recognised as being capable of rape, ie. they are old enough to be responsible for their actions. *The* homosexual (as opposed to homosexual acts) has only existed as a status in law, sexology and medicine since the 1860s; the transvestite distinguished from the transsexual since the 1940s. It is only in the latter half of this century that the Victorian gynaecological limitation of 'proper' female sexual fulfilment in reproduction and motherhood, has been redefined in terms of clitoral, orgasmic pleasure. Since the 1950s, prostitution and male homosexuality have been partially decriminalised, censorship of obscene materials has been partially relaxed, the gay male age of consent lowered to 18 years of age, legal recognition given to a diversity of family forms (single-parent, same-sex parenthood by means of surrogacy or adoption) etc. Rape law has been modified to recognise rape within marriage and male-rape. Abortion has become popularly recognised, under qualifying conditions, as 'a woman's choice' and all manner of viable reproductive technologies developed and recognised in law. Such changes are contested, generally opposed in the absolute name of nature and/or religion but, even across the relatively brief span of post-war history, the changes, many of which have been dramatic, are tangible.

On the basis of such evidence, the sociological focus is inevitably on the social construction of sexualities set against the dominant natural sciences, eg. medicine, genetics and clinical psychology, and the common-sense emphasis on sexualities, as expressions of some biological or psychological drive or essence. *Essentialism* rests on the absolute assumptions referred to in the previous section, that what is culturally normal is biologically and genetically natural, 'God-given', and, by definition, 'right'. From an essentialist perspective, sexualities are immutable and fixed. Sexual 'deviations' that go against 'God's laws', are by definition, 'wrong' and 'unnatural', the result of some biological or psychological pathology. Essentialism is unconcerned with pursuing the causes of what is natural and normal (for example, no geneticist has sought to identify the heterosexual gene), but seeks explanations and treatments for all that are deviant and, it is thereby assumed, unnatural.

Throughout this century, however, since Freud (1977) first proposed that we are all born with an undifferentiated sex-drive, harnessed through personality development, essentialist reasoning has been in gradual retreat within the so-called 'pure' sciences. It is now conceded by most geneticists that the genetic origins of homosexuality, even when 'proved' (and all current claims are vigorously disputed), would do no more than predispose those affected to homosexuality. This is a predisposition which allows for countervailing social influences and, one must presume, the same reasoning would apply to those without the 'gay gene' and their possible negotiable predisposition towards heterosexuality (Hamer *et al*, 1993). Essentialist sciences are, themselves, socially constructed. We may refer to them as pure sciences, but their goals and practices, although strictly controlled in many respects, are not literally pure, for their agendas, practices and ethics are set by the prevailing values and conventions of their time. Hence, as with so many key and familiar terms and phrases, we should put 'pure' in quotation marks to indicate that it is not what it appears to be.

While 'pure' science has tended to weaken its resistance to social constructionist accounts of sexualities, common-sense, insofar as one can judge from opinion polls and other forms of attitudes research, has remained more resiliently essentialist. Common-sense knowledge is of necessity 'straightforward', 'definitive' and 'taken-for-granted'. It is what 'everyone knows', whether in the 'collective consciousness' or arising out of some inner personal or 'sixth sense', as evidenced by familiar truisms: 'it's only natural that . . .'; 'the main purpose of sex is procreation, otherwise the human race would die out'; 'I don't care what you say it's disgusting, doing things with their bodies not intended by nature'. This is the knowledge of the unquestionable by the unquestioning, wary and mistrustful of 'experts' 'what do *they* know?' (Marquet *et al*, 1996), unless that is, *they* are 'real' scientists (men in white coats, working in laboratories) who 'prove' common knowledge to have been right all along.

Common-sense confirms the rules by which people live as fixed by forces out of their own control. It gives certainty and comfort about the inevitability of our way of life, at the core of which is the 'norm of marriage, the family and procreation . . . (which) provides (our) 'particular regime of truth'' (Mort, 1980). Around this 'regime of truth' circle degrees of sexual deviation, from relatively modest heterosexual misdemeanours, such as single parenthood and adultery, through the deeply immoral, but partially legal, such as adult-consenting homosexuality and prostitution 'in private', to the immoral and criminal, such as rape and paedophilia. The more deviant, the further outside the 'moral community', the more 'unnatural' the depiction of the protagonists, so that rapists and paedophiles are portrayed as pathologically so. The more conformist the more one's conformity is used as evidence of the power of 'nature'. Under such blind convictions the social, economic and political construction of sexualities proceed apace, unnoticed, indeed all the more efficiently because we lower our guard, not recognising the formative power of the sexual 'knowledge' we can hardly fail to take-in.

Although marriage, family and procreation provide our 'regime of truth', common-sense has much to say about other 'natural' aspects of sexualities that have significant gender inequalities as consequences. Men naturally have 'sex needs', genital in focus, are stronger and more sexually assertive. They respond more readily than women to pornographic stimuli and, once roused, require 'release'. Women are more emotional in their needs, more diffuse in their physiological responses, sexual fulfilment is properly found in settled relationships rather than acts (McIntosh, 1978). Within the past thirty or so years, the sexual needs of women have undergone a dramatic transformation away from reproduction and motherhood to physical fulfilment. This has been interpreted as the result of uncovering what has physiologically always been present, rather than the product of significant socio-economic changes. For both men and women, however, sexuality is still represented as physically and emotionally complementary and maturely fulfilled within stable, 'loving', heterosexual, procreative relationships.

Sexual excitement is in itself, outside the emotional ballast of relationships, 'raw nature' and is dangerous because likened to 'losing control', being 'out of it', 'we couldn't help ourselves', 'it was meant to happen'; typical euphemisms that remove responsibility from the actors involved and place it squarely on the animal within us, which surfaces when we are most aroused. It is simply common-sense that, when we are engaged in sexual acts, we are at our least restrained. Indeed, one of the great problems in much sexual health education is how to convey rational knowledge about, for example, safe-sex practices, when sexual arousal and excitement are culturally defined as being by definition irrational and unscripted?

Common-sense is nothing if not ambiguous. There are proverbs and sayings for all circumstances and, although predominantly essentialist, they are not necessarily so. For the many which mystify the natural by referring to: 'fate', 'sexual chemistry', 'eyes locking across crowded rooms', 'goose bumps', 'falling apart inside', 'love at first sight', 'basic instincts' and 'fatal attractions', there are some which bring us back to our sense of responsibility, albeit after the event: 'you made your bed, now lie on it'. This could apply to many unwanted effects, such as pregnancies or STD infections. As with so many aspects of contemporary sexualities, however, it is HIV and AIDS that provide the most graphic examples: 'many citizens of the so-called 'mainstream (heterosexual) population', lay people and politicians alike, consider the disease (AIDS) self-inflicted' (Pollak, 1992). Even bleak judgments, such as ' you've made your bed . . .' etc. are ambiguous about responsibility, often implying not so much rationally pursued self-destruction as lack of control of sexual arousal, especially when applied to minorities, such as gay men, bisexuals and IV users, all of whom, by being innately deviant or unnatural, are by definition it is reasoned, less controlled, sexually more voracious, 'promiscuous' than heterosexuals.

Common-sense essentialism reassures general populations that prevailing sexual norms are 'right'. AIDS appears as a dread warning leading politicians to reiterate 'family' or 'Victorian values' and the media to mobilise 'moral panics' around the 'deviants' concerned. Conversely, for the sexual 'deviants' themselves, essentialist explanations are also reassuring. They also remove from them, or severely reduce, their own responsibility for their actions, enabling them to minimise or deny the contamination threat they pose to conventional society. Paedophiles find little solace in such reasoning and claim instead, as do their social and medical controllers, that they may change over time with appropriate treatment. Popular reasoning is not, however, convinced, as recent local resistance movements to the return of convicted paedophiles into 'the community' after serving their sentences, demonstrate. By contrast, male homosexuals and lesbians have increasingly resorted to an essentialist explanation of their 'condition', claiming that, if they are biologically what they are, how can they lead astray or convert those who are biologically normal? Why should they, therefore, not be allowed to teach openly as 'gay'. They cannot influence their pupils towards homosexuality, except that is, those who have the genetic predisposition to be so.

With regard to the specific issues of sexual health and healthcare, which take up the bulk of this volume, it is important to note that, as with sociologists' criticisms of biological scientists, blinkered pursuit of the causes of unnatural, because deviant, sexual types, and of common-sense's equally blinkered judgmental essentialism, research into sexual health and healthcare treatments can only be properly undertaken if practitioners remove themselves as far as possible from the value-laden cultural environments in which they work. This is, of course, by no means easy. It is hardly surprising that fundamental common-sense essentialism has been reinforced through the crude rhetoric of AIDS-expressing fear, panic, doom-laden predictions, medical helplessness accompanied by graphic depictions of bodies wracked by the virus. But, as the final pages of this chapter will demonstrate, the AIDS experience of the past fifteen years, once past the initial paralysing panic stage, has been one of rapid advance for constructionist reasoning within medical research and healthcare. It recognises the ways in which specific sex acts, patterns of sexual behaviours and norms, are the result of social and cultural influences, not fixed natural drives, as manifest by the success in the social *re*construction of sexual lifestyles of informed 'at risk' populations. 'The public health achievements of the gay 'community' have been extraordinary' (Bloor, 1995: quoting Coxon and Carbello, 1989). In popular discourses, however, AIDS is the threatening social exception that proves the rule. It is a hiatus in the routines of sexual cultures which, despite the speedy 'rational' responses of some sexual populations, medical researchers and health care specialists, has generally been embraced as reassuring proof of the correctness of 'nature', and the dire consequences of ignoring that this is so.

To claim that sexualities are socially constructed is not to claim that such construction is straightforward and reducible to a basic set of clear-cut precepts, but to draw attention to the multiple ways in which sexualities are socially organised and discussed, in a culture still largely asserting that sexualities are determined by non-social forces. In the final section of this chapter, AIDS will be used as the exemplar healthcare issue which demonstrates the dynamic social reconstruction of sexualities. First, however, it is necessary to explain the sociological meaning of 'social construction' a little more fully.

The social construction of sexualities

To make sense of sexualities, we clearly need to look beneath all forms of essentialism, including common-sense, in order to identify the social institutions and power relations out of which they are forged. The key questions are not ' what is unnatural' or 'why', but:

- 'why are these the questions most frequently asked'
- 'what impact do these persistent questions have on the ways in which people think and act sexually'
- 'what other meanings exist to describe and rationalise specific sexual acts and those associated with them'
- 'what are the effects of these meanings on the ways in which individuals organise their sexual lives?' (Weeks, 1995)
- 'what are the effects of these meanings on the ways in which mainstream institutions including medical institutions, their 'experts' and 'practitioners', deal with populations so sexually defined'
- 'if the meanings are changed or influenced by the intervention of authoritative directives, for example through changes to sex laws or 'safe-sex' guidelines, what are the behavioural consequences'
- specifically in the context of this chapter and volume: 'What are the implications for differential sexual health promotion, care and treatment of social constructionist evidence set against essentialist?'

Answers require an assessment of the legal, political and economic contexts which formally structure and monitor people's lives. Before these **macro**social issues can be considered, however, it is necessary to consider smaller scale **micro**social questions, such as 'how do we, as sexual beings, interact in our everyday lives' and 'how do we negotiate with sexual 'knowledge' to the extent that the patterns of our sexual behaviours, and our sexual identities may change as we move through life?' Many of these questions were stimulated by the findings of the two Kinsey reports (Kinsey et al, 1948; 1953), which shocked with their findings on patterns of male and female human sexual behaviours. Kinsey was a biologist, not a sociologist, intent on discovering what he believed to be the universal patterns of sexual behaviour, and he produced a mountain of data which can be found summarised in a number of excellent secondary sources (Plummer, 1975; McIntosh, 1968; McIntosh, 1978; Hawkes, 1996). For our purposes, it is sufficient to note that, in one respect in particular, these studies, although biological in origin, raised questions which only sociologists could answer. In brief, it was clear that neither males nor females can be discretely categorised, as commonly assumed, as either hetero- or homosexual. Rather, their findings required the use of a seven-point continuum stretching from 100% heterosexuality at one end to 100% homosexuality at the other. The five inner points identified degrees of hetero- *and* homosexuality, or as is now preferred, degrees of bisexuality.

Kinsey was basically interested in 'outlets' (orgasms) and psychosexual attraction. With respect to the former, it was found that '37% of the male population has some homosexual experience between the beginning of adolescence and old age'; '25% of males had 'more than incidental' homosexual experiences for at least three years between ages 16 and 55, 18% being more homosexual than heterosexual for three consecutive years within the same age range' (Kinsey *et al*, quoted McCaffrey 1972).

The actual percentages are questionable due to weaknesses in the reserach methods used, but there is no doubting two overall findings: first that for a substantial proportion of men and women, sexual orientation and acts are not simply either hetero- or homosexual and second the pattern of behaviours and orientations of individual men and women may also change over time. Kinsey did not survey the rationales or explanations of his respondents but his findings clearly required that such research be carried out. The two major researchers to embark on this quest were initially trained as psychologists and employed to analyse the Kinsey data, out of which they developed what is known as the 'symbolic interactionist' approach to sexuality (Gagnon, 1967; Gagnon and Simon, 1967; 1970; 1973; 1986), subsequently further developed by others (Plummer, 1975) and now called simply 'interactionist'. These terms may appear daunting but the perspective is easily understood as long as one remembers that it uses a theatrical metaphor as will be demonstrated shortly.

These writers asserted their terms of engagement with some vigour:

> *'the sexual may be precisely that realm wherein the superordinate position of the socio-cultural order over the biological level is most complete.'*
>
> (Gagnon and Simon, 1973)

> *'sexuality is subject to socio-cultural moulding to a degree surpassed by few other forms of human behaviour.'*
>
> (Gagnon and Simon, 1973)

> *'nothing is sexual but naming it makes it so. Sexuality is a social construction learnt with others.'*
>
> (Plummer, 1975)

'An identifiable (sociological) approach dates from this period.'

(Vance, 1988).

Given the weight of essentialist opinion about human sexual behaviours, even in the social sciences, it should be added that: '... the struggle to move away from essentialist and naturalizing ways of thinking about sexuality has been a difficult one' (Vance, 1988).

'Interactionists' concentrate on **micro**social aspects of sexual life and learning, emphasising the dynamic everyday **emergence** of sexual identities, meanings, choices and preferences etc. arising out of the **negotiations** made by actors in interaction with others in different contexts. This may seem both dense and abstract, hence the value of deploying a theatrical metaphor. We are all actors who move through different stages (situations) in our everyday lives: home, train, bus, office, canteen, bus, train, home, pub, club, etc. On all these stages we use the scripts we have learnt, but we do not use the same scripts in all situations and, in any one situation we have room for interpretation and improvisation (negotiation) depending on the performances of the other actors present. These performances and scripts are not necessarily sexual, of course, but given our 'bio-power' obsessions, all actors are at all times sexual actors, and there is always a sexual presence in all performances. 'The individual learns to be sexual as he or she learns sexual scripts, scripts that invest actors and situations with erotic content' (Gagnon and Simon, 1969). At home we may be intimately acting with our gay lover, on the bus we may conceal or reveal our sexual identities by wearing badges or adopting coded dress codes, at work we may prefer to be 'closeted' and pretend to have a heterosexual lifestyle, although close friends might be told.

Potentially, this perspective might suggest that we are all hyperactively engaged in a very unstable world, but, in practice, we and the world are stabilised by the influence of norms and conventions, by the effects of routine in our daily lives, and our commitment to our own fixed sexual identities and lifestyles ('homosexual', 'bisexual', 'prostitute' etc). These scripts are primarily common-sense and mundane, and although such terms as **negotiation** and **emergence** imply conscious, rational and systematic thought and action, most of our interactions are carried out semi-consciously as a result of routine and familiarity. Within all interactions, however, everything or anything can have sexual meanings attached to them. In other words sexual meanings are not limited to the intrinsic qualities of an actor, act or object. Acts and objects can only be sexual if actors ascribe sexual meanings to them. Thus a book may be pornographic to some, 'high art' to others. A touch, friendly to some, harrassment to others, an unthinking aside may be full of sexual innuendo to some but undetected by others.

The implications for those who have to act in situations within which distinct sexual subcultural scripts operate are clear. Perform only with your heterosexual scripts in a gay situation with gay, lesbian or bisexual actors, and the interaction will soon break-down. Similarly, interpreting the actions of others, without regard to their own beliefs and rationalisations, will mean critically misunderstanding their meaning, not making sense of them. For example, a sex act between two men may be interpreted as 'homosexual' by one of them, merely 'release' to the other. This may prove shocking to some, how can the anal penetration of one man by another **not** be considered homosexual by one or both participants? Very possibly when the term 'homosexual' is severely stigmatised and is still, in many instances, stereotypically associated with effeminacy. The stigma of being gay can lead to lengthy life-time negotiations with identifying one's self as such, perhaps at the same time as one is married and a father. Similarly, if homosexuality is equated with effeminacy in men, males who are in all other respects conventionally masculine may interpret sex with other men as a sign of their general virility. In certain institutional settings, such as prisons, the two actors may both interpret their behaviour as primarily forced on them by the constraints of the setting, rather than by their sexual interests or orientations, believing that they will revert to heterosexuality once released. Such varied possibilities have become more familiar in the post-AIDS era by demonstrating the complex range of meanings a single sex act may have to the participants. Of course, the likelihood is that both men will define the act and themselves as 'homosexual' or, given the more positive implications of the term, 'gay', but they need not and if they do not the likelihood is that they will not in any other respect participate in a gay lifestyle or subculture. Rather than being labelled as homosexuals, it would be more accurate to describe them as men who have sex with other men. Clearly, we cannot make sense of sexuality unless we understand the varieties of meanings employed by all of us as sexual actors in such microsocial interactions.

Whatever the valuable sociological insights of the interactionist perspective, it has its shortcomings. As is evident, it is preoccupied with the study of interactions in small-group or institutional settings (such as prisons, schools, bars etc) and, as a result, the wider social context tends to be ignored, so that sexuality remains detached from formal social, political and economic structures and power relations of modern societies. Yet it is obvious that sexualities are integrated into these structures and relations: laws define the conditions of family life and illegal sex acts, and various officers enact these laws from tax inspectors and social workers to the police and magistrates. Meanwhile, sex is also sold as a commodity in its own right as well as being used subtly, and not so subtly, to sell anything else. So, while we do all use sexual scripts as sexual actors in our everyday interactions, we and our scripts are significantly constructed out of the macro-structures in which we are located. The example of the two men referred to earlier might demonstrate this in many ways. They might be having sex in a policed and thus dangerous 'public' space; their class, ethnic and religious identities will affect their interpretations of what they are doing. While interactionism is important for demonstrating that in our daily encounters sexualities are not innately fixed, it draws our attention away from the wider social and economic environment. Scripts are largely divorced from the power relations of wider society. It is also guilty of making us appear more conscious and in control of our actions than we actually are as the alternative approach of Michel Foucault (1981) makes clear.

Interactionists refer to scripts, Foucault prefers discourses. In a general sense they are the same: forms of sexual 'instruction' or 'knowledge'. But for Foucault, discourses are not power neutral scripts, rather they are weighed down by the inherent power they carry. He talks of the 'discursive explosion' which has elaborated all aspects of sexualities since the late nineteenth century and, at great length, about the roles of 'experts' in disseminating this 'knowledge'. We buy and read guides to sex, we read sexperts in newspapers, we confess to doctors or psychiatrists who feed us with analysis and cures etc, but these are especially keen to jolt us into recognising the power inherent in the seemingly trivial. Whereas interactionism implies we actively and consciously discriminate between and interpret scripts, Foucault claims that the most powerful and persuasive sexual discourses are precisely those we take-for-granted as being unimportant. The result is that we passively soak them up and become colonised by them, and when we express opinions and give meanings we are merely mouthing back all that we have learned.

Foucault places greatest emphasis on informal discourses: gossip, humour innuendo, and it is vital to remember that all of these cultural forms are full of powerful constraints on what we do and how we explain what we do. However, it is clear that we are also constrained by formal laws, moral guidance and the dictates of market forces. We are not actors in a power vacuum, nor are we merely passive dupes, completely unable to resist. The odds may be stacked against us far more than interactionism allows, but we remain social actors forced at times to make and justify consciously our choice of actions, partly because the discourses we encounter tell us different things. The government may tell us that certain sex acts and lifestyles are dangerous and/or illegal, but commercial interests may seek to sell the very same acts and lifestyles. Government agencies may seek to inform the public about 'safe-sex' but our reaction will depend upon our religious or ethnic beliefs, our age, social class, gender and sexual identities. In this context it is especially notable how, in the past thirty or so years, governments have consistently made pronouncements and introduced legislation confirming the validity and defence of traditional, Christian sexual values, thereby earning the epithet of the 'moral state'. Obscene materials, prostitution, homosexuality, single parenthood, child sex abuse, sex education are just a few of the battleground issues around which the 'moral state' raises the barricades. Simultaneously, it is also notable how leisure and lifestyle consumerism have consistently placed market pressures on these moral and legal constraints covering what can be legitimately sold and marketed. How they have exploited us into demanding such commodities, even on the black-market if necessary. With sufficient money one can purchase illegal obscene materials, obtain IV fertilisation treatments to obtain 'designer' babies, obtain late terminations to pregnancies, undergo transsexual surgery, if not in Britain then elsewhere.

For these reasons it may be argued that, although we are subjected to the 'moral' directives of the state, we are at the same time tempted into 'amoral' markets. This fundamental tension affects all aspects of sexual life. They induce dilemmas for us as actors, who are then forced to negotiate our way through the inherent contradictions, whatever our sexual identities and behavioural patterns. And it makes no difference whether we are patients/clients or practitioners in the sphere of sexual health and healthcare. In particular, it is clear that this tension has become increasingly organised and managed through the machinery and processes of citizenship.

Sexual citizenship

In Britain and other developed societies, the 1950s and 1960s were a period of unprecedented legal reform, affluence and burgeoning consumerism. Sexuality was incorporated as an 'autonomous sphere of pleasure and self-expression, with its own intrinsic value and justification . . . in the context of mutual consent and respect' (Seidman, 1989). In other words, it was in this period that sexual pleasure for its own sake became a legitimate goal within the expanding leisure industry. The most significant legal document of this 'era of the legislation of consent' (Hall, 1979), *The Wolfenden Report* advocated that the law should draw a distinction between 'private (sexual) morality' and 'public good', between crime and sin, as follows:

> *'... it is not the function of the law to interfere in the private lives of citizens, or to seek to enhance any particular pattern of behaviour'*
>
> (*The Wolfenden Report*, 1957)

Yet it was/is still the law's duty to:

> *'preserve public order and decency . . . protect the citizen from what is offensive and injurious . . . and provide safeguards against the exploitation and corruption of others . . . Unless a deliberate attempt is made by society, acting through the agency of the law, to equate the sphere of crime with that of sin, there must remain a realm of private morality and immorality which is not the law's business.'*
>
> (*The Wolfenden Report*, 1957)

The recommended change in legal emphasis was from moral to causal judgments so that acts were not to be judged on the basis of whether they were morally 'wrong' but whether they had bad effects: 'if it turns out that more harm is done by forbidding an activity than by allowing it, then Parliament will permit it, even if most of the members consider that activity to be wrong or immoral' (Davies, 1975). The association of illegality with immorality was severed, and between their boundaries a social, economic and political space was created for those which were justly legalised but still morally reprehensible. Male homosexuals and female prostitutes were the test-cases specified on the grounds that whatever the moral considerations, their participants were largely consenting adults and, if properly monitored, their effects on the rest of society, minimal. It was not intended to remove or weaken the stigma of immorality. Wolfenden described homosexuality as 'reprehensible from the point of view of harm to the family' (Wolfenden, 1957) and emphasised that public manifestations of prostitution and homosexuality should be severely policed. However, a legal/immoral 'space' was created for all deemed legal but immoral who, as a result, acquired distinct citizenship rights and responsibilities, a geographical mainly urban space (Bell and Valentine, 1995), outside and 'around the norm of marriage, the family and procreation' (Mort, 1980).

While the legal retreat from immorality on grounds of 'consent' and 'privacy' has become the norm, it is still contested. Nor is there a complete absence of legislation which readdresses the link between sin and crime. In response to a question posed by *The Times* (January 14th, 1994): 'Is it part of the state's task to regulate sexual behaviour', Oxford Law Professor, John Finnis claimed: 'A political community that judges that the stability and educative generosity of family life is of fundamental importance, can rightly judge that it has a compelling interest in doing whatever it can to discourage (homosexual) conduct', effectively the intent of *Section 28* of *The Local Government Act* (1988). But in so claiming, Finnis ignored the crucial complication already referred to, namely that 'moral' state policies on sexual citizenship and the law have an ambiguous relationship with 'amoral' market pressures to enhance commercial exploitation of immoral and illegal sexual populations through the sale of profitable sexual commodities.

As this account of categories of sexual citizenship demonstrates, liberal assumptions on citizenship are misplaced. One such is provided by Aristotle as follows:

- 'citizens . . . are all who share in the civic life of ruling and of being ruled' (Aristotle, 1972)
- having the right to be consulted on the conduct of the political society 'and the duty of having something to contribute to the general consultation',
- being 'bound by the results . . . for duties flow from . . . rights' (Brogan, 1960).

This model of citizenship consists of idealised inclusionary principles, of a respectful, contractual relationship between autonomous, moral subjects and their state. In practice, however, sexual citizenship has developed as elaborate tariffs of partial or complete exclusion according to sexual status and moral conformity, as inspection of the famed accounts of Rawls (1972; 1987) and Marshall (1950) unintentionally, make clear.

Rawls (1987) is the more complex, and baffled readers should perhaps move swiftly to Marshall three paragraphs on, but Rawls is a central contemporary analyst and citizenship issues *are* complex. He identifies as fundamental to citizenship rights, the social and natural primary goods which any rational person would want 'whatever (their) social orientation'. Social primary goods include 'the basic liberties' such as freedom of thought and liberty, freedom of movement and choice of occupation where there are diverse opportunities, the powers and prerogatives of offices and positions of responsibility which 'give scope to various self-governing and social capacities of the self', income and wealth and all social bases of self-respect. In all, those aspects of basic institutions are essential 'if citizens are to have a lively sense of their own worth as persons and be able to develop and exercise their moral power and advance their aims with self-confidence'. Natural primary goods include health and vigour, intelligence and imagination.

Rawls (1972) locates these primary goods in specific social contexts according to 'principles of justice' which rest on the most extensive justifiable set of equal basic liberties for all, social and economic inequalities, roles and offices, open to all under conditions of 'fair equality of opportunity'. Rawls locates such principles and practices of 'justice' in a particular society's economic, political and other institutions where rights and duties are assigned and monitored, and a 'citizenship culture' is established in which 'the legitimate expectations' of populations are accepted as given and/or through which claims of injustices in rights and state practices are challenged.

The net effect of this analysis, however, is that citizenship becomes potentially restrictive on particular subjects. Rawls' notions of 'self-confidence', 'sense of self-worth', 'plan of life', 'scope for self-government', the realisation and expression of 'social capacities of the self', etc, are not universally inclusive, but depend upon qualifying conditions, such as conformity to mainstream sexual norms of behaviour and 'orientation'. Non-conformity justifies a lesser sense of self-worth, a restricted 'plan of life' less 'scope for self-government' etc.

In addition, Rawls links 'egalitarian' principles of justice to differential market access, wealth and income, as part of 'legitimate expectations', affirming a relationship now enshrined in Britain in the *Citizen's Charter* (Department of Health, 1991). So a causal relativism is implicit in liberal accounts of citizenship. Full membership depends on conformity to conventions, and once such a principle is established, the history of citizenship consists of battles over the legitimacy of **relative** claims to rights and resources, within which health, a natural right of justice for Rawls, is inevitably implicated. It must also be stressed that such claims within a 'liberal' citizenship culture depend on acceptance by claimants of their common stigmatised status, set against the morality of the dominant sexual order and the relative illegitimacy of their claims to 'equality' because 'unnatural'.

As acknowledged above, drawing such conclusions from a brief account of Rawls work is possibly complex and baffling, but Marshall's (1950) account is much more accessible. His analysis of citizenship in the capitalist era as an evolutionary democratisation of **civil**, through **political** to **social** rights, also explains the legitimacy of discriminatory disqualification against 'minority' (sexual) status groups, by, for example, describing social rights as: 'the right to share to the full in the social heritage and . . . live the life of a civilised being *according to the standards prevailing in the society* (my italics). While all citizens of democracies may be 'free and equal persons' in a general sense (Rawls 1987), the state's protection of 'standards prevailing in the society' requires and justifies differential, limited citizenship for those who might threaten these standards.

Thus drawing on the *Wolfenden* legal watershed and such models of liberal citizenship, conventional sexual standards are protected by two lines of defence; the inner one moral, the outer one legal, which specify two broad constellations of 'deviant' sexual citizens outside the 'moral community'. Beyond the outer line of defence, are those deemed both criminal **and** immoral: convicted paedophiles, rapists, sado-masochists, purveyors and users of hard-core pornography etc, who forfeit their 'free' citizenship status until the terms of their sentence have been served, and who even then have a 'record' justifying yet more severe punishment if found guilty of reoffending. Within this outer defensive line of illegality, but outside the 'moral community' is located a second, larger, category of sexual citizens, conditionally 'legal' but resolutely immoral: homosexuals, bisexuals, lesbians, transvestites, transsexuals, prostitutes etc. These populations are 'legal' as long as deference is paid to qualifying conditions which, if disregarded, can lead to relegation into the criminal category, conditions which, although specific to the particular minority addressed, commonly require citizens of this type to confine 'open' expression of their 'immoral' sexual statuses — behaviour, dress, political demands, media coverage — to 'private' or 'semi-private' settings to avoid offending the 'moral community'. Gay men who have sex in public places, such as parks, toilets and beaches, and street-working prostitutes are the most common transgressors. In effect, the illegal and immoral are policed formally into 'privacy', while the legal yet immoral are expected to police themselves into a 'privacy' monitored by the police proper at the boundaries.

Conformity to these conditions has been rewarded with the gradual development of distinct, although reduced, rights and responsibilities compared to those enjoyed by the moral and legal. Members of the 'moral community' are assumed to be effectively policing themselves unless exposed as otherwise, in which case relegation may place them into either of the other two categories, depending on the extent of 'deviation' revealed.

These three categories of sexual citizenship: (i) legal and moral: (ii) legal yet immoral: (iii) illegal and immoral, affect not only the norms and lifestyles, but present particular challenges to those in mainstream 'moral' society who interact with them, including those engaged in sexual health promotion, care and treatment. For example, official recognition that a significant proportion of same-sex prison populations who do not define themselves as homosexual, are actively sexual is highly problematic and rarely forthcoming (Gagnon and Simon, 1968). Targeting male homosexuals may work most effectively through the gay media by using sub-cultural terms which explicitly describe sexual practices, terms invariably deemed 'offensive' to and in 'the moral community'. However, many men who have sex with men are beyond the reach of such targeting methods. They may be infrequent participants in specifically gay territories, never buy gay magazines, only frequent 'outside cruising' areas and, as in the earlier example, may not identify as 'gay'.

Like the latter, prostitutes who solicit 'in public' technically break the law, but rigid and rigorous law enforcement also drives them further out of reach of health care agencies. Meanwhile, in mainstream 'moral' culture where sexuality is surrounded by secrecy and embarrassment, effective sex education and instruction, especially for those still at school, becomes fraught with tensions and conflicts over parental, children's and teacher's rights, leading more often than not to simple avoidance, ignorance, confusion and distress. But, as has been noted, citizenship is not solely a matter of packages of political rights and duties, it is also directly implicated in economic rights, market access and participation through which the common lifestyles of specific status groups are expressed.

> '... status groups are normally communities ... determined by a specific positive or negative social estimation of honour ... which always rests upon distance and exclusiveness ... normally expressed by the fact that above all else a specific style of life can be expected from all those who wish to belong to the circle.'
>
> (Weber, 1967)

Sexual status groups are not merely part-time 'communities' defined by differential political and civil rights and duties appropriate to their relative moral honour or esteem, they also develop distinctive consumption lifestyles in which:

> '... consumer conduct (becomes) the cognitive and moral focus of life, integrative bond of society ... individuals are (now) engaged (morally by society, functionally by the social system) first and foremost as consumers rather than producers'
>
> (Bauman, 1988)

The consumer and the drive to consume have a great deal in common with the sexual subject's will to 'know' more and more about their sexualities. As consumers we also believe we are 'unique' individuals with personalities expressed through the commodities we buy. So, to return to an earlier observation, if 'sexuality has become the medium through which people seek to define their personalities and to be conscious of themselves' (Foucault and Sennett, 1981), the search and self, are in great measure going to be in the form of commodities consumed. If our sexual identities are the deepest reality with which it is our duty to come to terms, then we must come to terms with not only sex acts, dysfunctions, *the Big O* (Heath, 1982), health, pleasure and happiness, but also with the purchase of appropriate lifestyles. If 'Reality as the consumer experiences it is the pursuit of pleasure (Featherstone, 1988) as 'on display we move through the field of commodities' in 'search of personal and private satisfactions above all else' (Hobsbawm, 1981), the latter are increasingly sexual, their realisation forged out of material circumstance. The parallels are strong and no coincidence. The pursuit of the commodified self is the pursuit of the sexual self; both dressed up as our need to find our 'unique' 'essence', conspicuously enacted through the acquisition and expression of particular goods and the styles of life they are associated with, by populations who differentially qualify as citizens according to their conformity to 'standards prevailing in society'.

Appropriate as such a model of differential sexual citizenship may be, its usefulness depends on the recognition of at least four complications:

1. These are not three formally fixed, discrete categories. 'Deviant' sexual status is often concealed in at least some social settings where heterosexual normality is assumed, unless revealed through self-disclosure or exposure by others, and 'criminal' sexual status is in many respects notoriously hard to investigate and prove.

2. Nor are the legal and moral lines of defence around the 'moral community' fixed and static. Like all lines of defence, both are also lines of attack, with constant battles over matters of sexual decriminalisation and rights advances, often waged on behalf of those excluded, by groups within. There are numerous current or recent examples. A significant proportion of 'presumed to be straight' MPs supported the unsuccessful attempt to reduce the gay male age of consent to 16 years in the Commons 'free' vote of February 1994. The Chief Constable of West Yorkshire police, Keith Hellawell is but one senior officer who has called for the legalisation of brothels (*The Independent*, July 29th 1996) to 'get women off the streets and to more effectively safeguard their health'. Lord Hope, the most senior judge in Scotland, endorsed in July 1996 the first case of adoption (of a five-year old mentally and physically disabled child) in the United Kingdom by a gay male who 'has lived in a close and loving relationship with another man for ten years' (*The Times*, July 27th 1996).

3. As these examples imply, within each of these three categories of sexual citizen there are further fine degrees of 'deviance' and, in effect, fine degrees of sexual health and ill health: teenage girls frightened because, or perhaps unaware that, they are pregnant, single mothers of any age, those who use potentially dangerous sex toys, women who after fertility treatment become pregnant with eight foetuses, 'open marriages', promiscuous gay men, part-time 'masseuses' etc.

4. It has to be reiterated that, although specific rights battles of the kind referred to above may be explicitly fought and sexual status groups and identities acknowledged, generally, our sexual culture is one in which sexual knowledge is learned and exchanged in indirect ways. We may be increasingly obsessed by and 'knowledgeable' about the sexual, but our obsessions remain largely refracted, our 'knowledge' euphemistic rather than explicit. This means that we find it particularly difficult as researchers or professional practitioners to act and rationalise in non-judgmental and discriminatory ways. With these qualifications, this model of sexual citizenship provides the dimensions of the macrosocial construction of sexualities, and within which the micro interactions take place.

Sexual citizenship and dimensions of sexual health

To make sense of sexualities is to recognise that inside the 'moral community' is where conventional heterosexuality is integrated into all aspects of social life. Unconventional sexual populations consist of 'constituencies' with distinct sets of rights and duties, rather than 'communities' as such, because membership is, at best, part-time and mainly limited to leisure activities (Coxon and Carbello, 1989[1]). Each 'constituency' participates in distinct subcultures, although within the gay 'constituency', there are numerous sub-affiliations and interests. Sexual health concerns vary for each of these subgroups, as does their accessibility to researchers and healthcare workers, and the willingness of members to seek healthcare and treatment and to be 'open' about their sexual life histories with healthcare workers. This is especially so for those on the outskirts of each 'constituency' and those with 'illegal' interests and lifestyles. Accessing populations to deliver sexual health knowledge is not simply a matter of finding those targeted, but communicating with them in the appropriate language. For example, for those who frequent gay bars and clubs, the language has to be one which cuts through the idealised commercial imagery of sexual abandonment to be found in gay media, in which 'safety' messages find little emphasis. For those on the periphery, however, a style less directly implicating gay identity is probably required, while in the 'biopower' context effective sexual health information, care and treatment should extend beyond the narrow and explicit aspects of sexual health to wider lifestyles issues, such as drug and alcohol use and misuse.

Sexual health among the illegal and immoral, mainly although not exclusively those in prison, poses distinct problems for practitioners. But so, too, does the sexual health of many in the 'moral community' in which open and direct discussion of sexual issues is generally taboo. To efficiently transmit sexual health 'knowledge' under these circumstances is to risk being too explicit in terms and practices and, thereby, to cause offence. The constraining influence of this 'moral community' inevitably influences the health dimensions within both illegal/immoral and legal/immoral forms of sexual citizenship. Given that for more than a century, the male homosexual and female prostitute have served as the 'folk devils' through which heterosexual normality has been defined, given also that, through terms such as 'pouf' and 'tart', both serve as common-sense signposts for sexual impropriety and, finally, given that the greatest health concern of the past 15 years has been HIV transmission and AIDS, the concluding discussion will concentrate on these two 'constituencies'.

There are several key elements which have shaped the the ways in which social scientists and healthcare workers have dealt with HIV transmission and AIDS.

1. Initially and throughout the 1980s, there was a need to work more speedily than normal in scientific research and healthcare: 'How can one deal with the different aspects of AIDS-fear and stigmatisation of the infected, coping mechanisms, organisation of care and prevention — without adopting an attitude of intervention in a crisis?' The ideal balance between 'involvement' and 'detachment' was hard to achieve, especially as 'doing research was synonymous with being solicited to participate in practical work: educational sessions in healthcare units or in the first voluntary associations, organising hot lines and counselling services. Social work and social science research were intimately intertwined'. Speedy action also meant the making of culturally biased assumptions in the name of expediency (Pollak, 1992).

2. Given the speed and scale of the crisis, the established response was of organisational and intellectual inertia. Researchers had to quickly decide whether to change and risk careers, one result being a self-selection of young academics into research in this area and of young doctors and nurses to treat and care. Many of the latter acquired reputations as AIDS specialists in contrast to their low rank in the wider medical hierarchy. With increased ward case loads, conflicts with superiors were inevitable over the orientation and specialisation of hospital services, the number of beds and the paramedical personnel available for AIDS patients, given that . . .

3. . . . resources for social scientific research in the field of AIDS were scarce. 'AIDS arrived at a time of severe restrictions in public spending in most western countries' (Pollak, 1988).

4. Conventional defensive attitudes within 'the moral state' and 'moral community' delayed or made impossible large research projects dealing with sexuality:

> *In the United Kingdom . . . PM Margaret Thatcher (decided) that public research should not intrude into the private sphere of citizens. Without public funding the project took off a year later with private support from the pharmaceutical industry. But the public controversy had a decided effect on the response rate.*
>
> (Pollak, 1988)

Thatcher vetoed the initial draft of the Government's first anti-AIDS advertising campaign in 1986 for being like 'writings on a lavatory wall' (Evans, 1993). In 1988, a Jesse Helms' amendment was passed by the US Senate limiting educational and research programmes by excluding federal funds for projects that could encourage homosexual activities (Bayer, 1989), and *Section 28* has been similarly constraining in Britain, culturally and financially if not legally (Evans, 1989/90). Age of consent legislation limits access to those underage; parental authority rules also limit 'free' discussion. Research into the sexual behaviours and attitudes of those at school require special authorisation from administrators and parents. Generally hard to obtain, it becomes almost impossible if questions on same-sex contacts are included. Tourism heightens sexual activity and risk-taking, but 'safe-sex' campaigns at airports to counter 'sex and sun' summer holiday cultures have also met with considerable church and political opposition.

5. This relates to what Pollak calls 'sheer prejudice'. Often the hesitant response to AIDS has been due to its association with 'proximate causes': homophobia, discrimination and criminalisation of marginalised populations, such as intravenous drug users and a generally failing health policy and care sector.

> *. . . if there is some tolerance in society for marginal groups, there has been no willingness to change political and research agendas as long as AIDS was defined as primarily affecting stigmatized and increasingly poor groups. Many citizens of the . . . 'mainstream (heterosexual) population', lay people and politicians alike, consider the disease self-inflicted . . . the largest number of AIDS cases in the western world are still homosexual and bisexual males and IV drug users. By and large society rejects these forms of behaviour and consumption.*
>
> (Pollak, 1992)

Epidemiological writings still react with surprise and misunderstanding to numbers of sexual partners and sexual practices, illustrating 'the extent to which homosexuals and bisexuals are 'foreigners' to their neighbours and co-citizens' (Coxon, 1988; Watney, 1988, Rühmann, 1985).

6. The methodological difficulties of accessing specific populations are especially crucial (Siegel and Bauman, 1986; Zich and Temoshok, 1986). To be accepted, researchers have to prove their research will do no harm to the 'constituencies' they analyse: gay men, drug users, prostitutes and their clients. They have to acquire legitimacy without becoming transformed into movement spokespersons. The sexual preference of the researcher or practitioner need not necessarily be a 'passport' into fields of study, but for some it means having an enhanced subcultural awareness. McKeganey and Barnard, neither prostitutes I hasten to add, describe their 'access' route to street working prostitutes in Glasgow as:

> . . . necessitating the creation of an acceptable social role in order to be in the red-light area in the first place. With the agreement of the local health board and having informed the local police of what we intended to do, we adopted a quasi-service-provider role . . . providing women working on the streets with supplies of condoms, sterile injecting equipment, information on HIV risk reduction and phone numbers of . . . local services. Each night's fieldwork . . . consisted of walking round all the streets where sex was being sold, approaching as many women as possible, introducing ourselves, offering them the various items we were carrying. In this way we gradually became familiar to the women and this, in turn, facilitated the build-up of sufficiently good relationships with the women to allow the research to proceed.
>
> (McKeganey and Barnard, 1996)

The more privatised targeted populations, the harder they are to access: 'There is simply not enough information available on women working in off-street prostitution to be confident of the assertion that HIV is clustered among women working on the streets'. Like gay men, female and male prostitutes do not constitute a single unitary category:

> . . . the call man with his own flat and a 'book' of regular clients . . . is far removed from a crowd of jostling half-drunk adolescents milling around the steps of a late-night public lavatory. Among street working male prostitutes (some) have the same instrumental and businesslike orientation as their female

> *street-prostitute colleagues . . . others have a casual and haphazard approach . . . more in common with juvenile delinquency than female prostitution.*
>
> (Bloor, 1995)

Particular citizenship cultures also manifest specific negotiation strategies. The most common reasons for non-use of condoms by prostitutes include the practical: poor supplies and lack of confidence due to frequent failure, but extend to not using them with partners or spouses, to distinguish between sex for money and sex for love (Day, 1988). Also prostitute/client relationships are power relationships, hence non-condom use can be because 'punters' do not want to use them, or are prepared to pay more for sex without them. Sexual excitement is also associated with abandon, 'escape' including 'escape' from 'safe-sex' warnings, the abandonment of precautions. Indeed for many, sexual excitement is all the better for being dangerous and risky.

Research shows high levels of HIV transmission knowledge among men who have sex with men despite initial scepticism tinged with irony that gay men are encouraged to take instruction from 'the very same science that has sought to discipline our sexualities' (Woodhead, 1995). The heterosexual or bisexual self-identified are less well informed and less likely to practice 'safe(r) sex'. By not self-identifying as homosexual, and by rarely if ever placing themselves in gay 'constituency' territories they appear able to distance themselves from being 'at risk'.

Health work in peripheral territories, such as toilets and parks, tends to be carried out by volunteer-staffed groups such as GMFA (Gay Men Fighting AIDS) with varying degrees of co-operation from the police[2]. Radical health promotion, seeking to by-pass the bureaucratised practices of much official sexual health work, disseminates 'safe-sex' messages in a subcultural language which avoids the rhetoric of science and 'expert'. Such groups have, for some, 'legitimated sex between men in the forum of public health' (Woodhead, 1995), but this has not been without problems. A volunteer-led organisation may be more democratic than a professionally led one. But the volunteers, themselves, are unlikely to be representative of the whole 'constituency', coming as they do from a narrow, self-selecting already-aware sector, that has little or no contact with other men who might regard HIV as an issue in their lives. By being committed to a clearly defined 'community' approach, institutional recognition by funding bodies may be forthcoming, but, in the process, the latter may assume that all those in need are being successfully reached and their needs met, thus ignoring broad sections of the wider 'constituency'. The radical promise of such projects ultimately rests on the assumption that **out** gay men can somehow reflect the worries of all men who have sex with men. Although volunteer-staffed and with 'alternative' agendas, such organisations serve as power/knowledge disciplining forces every bit as pervasive as any formally employed by the state.

7. Pollak (1994) reports in some detail on the difficulties in eliciting accurate responses from respondents, no matter how questions are formulated, and how the respondents are found, the latter being clearly critical. For longitudinal purposes, cohort members are recruited, usually through health services, STD clinics or networks of gay doctors. These are atypical in their HIV status, openness about sexual matters and changed behaviours. Contacts with gay 'community' associations, media, etc. are also crucial. For example, recruitment of 741 male homosexuals in Amsterdam in 1984 was possible because of the relationship between the Municipal Health Service and the gay male 'community' during several epidemiologic and prevention studies of STDs (van Griensven, 1987). But evidence shows that men involved in cohort studies are predominantly single, professional and highly educated (Pollak, 1994), suggesting that class representative homo- and bisexual research samples are especially difficult to obtain because working-class and less educated males have a lower presence in the core 'gay scene' than their numbers would suggest. The 'scene' is increasingly commodified and commercialised, in short, expensive, modelled on middle-class values and lifestyles, and discouraging to working-class and ethnic minority males.

Different forms of access bring different biases in sample size and make-up. Inserting health questionnaires in gay magazines privileges people with 'a certain gay self-consciousness expressed in membership or readership of specialised organisations and media' (Pollak, 1994). Indeed the likely bias appears extreme. A 'gay scene' drug survey by *Gay Times* (September 1996) compared its **readershi**p response to that of a 1 in 10 sample drawn from London's 1996 Gay Pride Rally. In the readership sample, 63% earnt £26,000+ a year, compared with 15% of the Pride sample. Two percent of the former earned less than £5,000 compared to 29% of the latter. Forty-five percent and 28% of the readership respondents were in managerial/professional and skilled manual occupations compared with 19% and 9% of the Pride sample.

Snowball sampling — where researchers set up networks of collaborators at different locales to hand out a set number of questionnaires to men having sex with men, and ask the recipients of these questionnaires to encourage other male aquaintances and friends to do the same — also carries a middle-class bias. It is easier to distribute questionnaires in bars and clubs than in toilets. Quota sampling, which attempts to match the sociodemographic characteristics of the general population by age, profession, educational level and residence, also has problems at the peripheral class and ethnic extremes.

'Project Sigma', using sex diaries kept by respondents contacted through gay media, had disappointing responses from working-class and ethnic minority populations and, like all sex diaries as well as cohort studies, lost a significant number of respondents over time (Coxon, 1988). In countries where gay magazines have limited circulation and associations are small, distributing questionnaires in meeting places is the preferred means for recruiting large numbers of respondents, but the inevitable urban bias becomes problematic. GHA Survey Result's 1989 Eire study used this method, 44% of their respondents were contacted in Dublin bars with Dublin over-representation, especially for age groups: 20–29 and 30–39 years.

Because of their wide circulation, newspaper samples reach larger numbers but with other biases. In Denmark 2100 male homosexuals and bisexuals answered a questionnaire enclosed in two gay magazines in Autumn 1988, but 66% of respondents were members of the national gay and lesbian LBL (Schmidt, quoted Pollak, 1994). Usually only 12–15% of questionnaires distributed in this way are returned, a high proportion from those with strong political or associational affiliations, again more middle-class and with higher than average levels of education, living in the larger cities. It appears that access to gay magazines is, for the majority, spasmodic rather than regular, only 30% of French respondents were regular readers of *Gai Pied* with two segments of the gay population over-represented; the most self-identifying living in Paris, and the most isolated living in rural areas for whom *Gai Pied* formed their only relationship with the gay community (Pollak, 1988). Others, however, have found that gay paper surveys reach a higher proportion of those of lower socio-economic status than other sampling techniques (Bochow, 1990).

With these qualifications, all studies show the incidence of anal sex and number of sexual partners to have dramatically fallen, and condom use, incidences of solitary and mutual masturbation and the number of closed-couple relationships to have risen (Pollak 1994). However, it is the exceptions who are most worrying. Men who have sex with men, living in localities of less than 20,000, often hiding their sexual preference or their homosexuality and not accepted by family, colleagues and friends, fear discrimination arising out of 'exposure' as homosexual as much as HIV infection and AIDS. They have little solidarity with a gay group, their capacity for individual behavioural changes is limited and diffusion of condom use slow. Until the late 1980s, blue-collar men were hardly concerned with AIDS at all, lower middle-class gays in the big cities (service sector) showed the highest degree of denial. Although well-informed about the disease, they often presented the 'risk-group' classification as an attempt to discriminate against them. Their biographical background, often including breaking up with their family because of being gay, explains their ambivalent reactions in the early days of the epidemic. Higher professionals and the more highly educated were the first to change behaviours, to know someone HIV+ or who had AIDS. The first volountary gay health self-help groups formed to combat AIDS, were self-recruited from this latter population.

There are striking national differences. In Germany, France and Ireland, regular condom use in anal penetration has become a gay habit, in Switzerland and Holland there has been a massive abandonment of anal penetration. Despite these changes, at the end of the 1980s there are reported levels of unprotected anal sex of 20% in France and 39% in the Netherlands, which could reflect an increase in monogamous partnerships where both partners are seronegative. In Amsterdam 68% of respondents have not taken the test, in Paris 30%. From the start, in Holland explicitness was paramount, including the push for a stronger condom for male anal penetrative use with appropriate water-soluble lubricants and 'jack-off parties', deemed crucial to learning 'safe sex' and where 'hot lines' guarantee anonymity. In Belgium, Norway and Spain 'love, tenderness and monogamy are mentioned as viable alternatives to an anonymous sex life' (Pollack, 1994). In some countries such measures are hampered by legal constraints, for example, in Eire where male homosexuality has only recently been legalised and in France where condom promotion was illegal until 1984. Britain has been without a central strategy and with little coordination between associations and public authorities, resulting in often contradictory and conflicting arguments. The Terence Higgins Trust and other gay-linked associations have argued for promotion of condoms; the government's 1986 campaign rested on 'Don't die of ignorance', with no practical guidance.

Statistical exercises are important but they can reify rigid sexual boundaries and population categories, so to correct any such impression it should be noted that on average 20–40% of samples of men who have sex with men have had sexual experiences with women (Pollak and Schiltz, 1991). Most 'bisexual' respondents have only one female partner and a much larger number of males, explained mainly because most practising bisexual men are married or divorced. The former usually have less male partners than the divorced, but are more likely to use condoms with male partners.

Unsurprisingly, 'social proximity to infected people induces the feeling of personal risk exposure and adopting low-risk behaviours ... reinforced by a level of social integration into a network of supportive groups and by the degree to which one's social environment accept homosexuality' (Pollak, 1994). Among men peripheral to such involvements and the young, the desire to experience and to fulfil a sexual need can overwhelm known dangers of unsafe sex (Prieur, 1990). Unsafe sex is engaged in for several reasons: the need for intimacy, to signal 'love', a sense of fatalism or no future. Three phases of negotiated broad responses in France have been noted: before 1985–86 the emergence of 'pioneers' practising safer sex, self-identified as gay and with high self-esteem, socially accepted and with confidence in medical authorities. Not individual 'pioneers', they reflected a middle-class professional, highly educated response. Between 1986–88, availability of the HIV test led especially informed groups to identify a collective risk and adopt new personal ethics of sexual precaution, which went beyond personal knowledge of someone infected to mobilisation of voluntary organisations. After 1988, there emerged recognition of the macrosocial limits of such a response: low socio-economic status, unemployment, low educational levels, low self-esteem, foreshortened expectations of life generally, sense of stigma, unacceptability to close kin or friends, experience of discrimination etc. For these, difficult to access anyway, personal counselling is considered of particular importance.

The author has left the reader to draw parallels between the substantive evidence in this section and the earlier theoretical analysis. It should be apparent that, for all the actors involved in the sequence of dramas with HIV and AIDS, there is constant renegotiation with discourses which are laden with moral and disciplinary power. Those who develop early symptoms of HIV-related illnesses are actors with already distinctive social identities through which these early inklings of ill health are filtered, perhaps with friends, perhaps with medical help, but in many cases alone. Becoming an AIDS patient is not simply a medical process but a tortuous reconstruction of one's whole identity with the sexual at its core, the long sought 'mystery' cruelly revealed. Such patients develop their own strategies for acquiring and dealing with AIDS 'knowledge'. In many cases, complex technical knowledge of the drugs they are or could be on, but also strategies of what is questionably called 'denial', the common-sense stigma of being a 'guilty' as opposed to 'innocent' victim, the fear, practical problems of living, maintaining an identity in the face of the medicalisation process in which what so often passes for 'denial' of being ill can be a 'denial' of the medical profession's right to control and deny patients' the rights to determine their own destinies in the name of 'care'. 'We have an oracle-client relationship, those with prescient or fore-knowledge and those lacking and in need of knowledge. Health promotion practices seek to discipline individuals through their surveillant discursive practices' (Woodhead, 1995) and, arguably, they do not only discipline but take the very 'identity' away from patients:

> *This plague has attracted the inevitable swarm of AIDS researchers, officials, businessmen, and journalists, and they are the ones who have monopolized the media. We people with AIDS, who devote every waking moment to our own survival, have been unable to prevent these loquacious experts from stealing our thunder and robbing us of the only thing we have left: our illness.*
>
> (Dreuilhe, 1987)

Those at risk of HIV infection have been shown to develop **selection** and **protection** negotiation strategies. The former include avoiding people (having fewer partners, because of their looks, their age or geographic origin), places (saunas or backrooms) and situations (alcohol or drug consumption), considered risky and likely to reduce self-control. **Protection** strategies involve changes in the acts engaged in. Initially, strategies were naively of the former kind: 'avoid American tourists', 'don't fuck with big city gays' etc (Pollak, 1994), which had little effect on the path or form of the epidemic. In the mid 1980s **protection** strategies became paramount. Subsequently, the availability of the HIV+ seropositivity test has led to informed strategies rather than 'guesswork' and the use of mixed strategies and differentiated risk-taking, such as no precautions with a steady partner in the case of a common seronegativity, safer sex with condoms with all casual partners. Even so, some, younger working-class males especially, may see HIV infection as a distant ten to fifteen year risk and, as such, hard to realistically contemplate. Working-class culture is marked by immediate rather than postponed aims and concerns, middle-class culture by deferred gratification. Hence sexual strategies are likely to be class as well as religion and ethnicity informed.

Professional healthcare workers also have to negotiate with all manner of discourses: common-sense judgments, their own as well as those of other actors with whom they deal, not least their 'clients'. They have to assess research developments, new drugs and alternative treatments, balancing their proven or claimed benefits against their often excessive costs, defending their decisions within a competitive health regime where the claims of sexual minorities in common with general citizenship criteria, are frequently judged of lower worth and, as the above comments by Woodhead and Dreuilhe indicate, there has to be negotiation with patients whose overall social make-up and identities should not be presumed and should be left intact. If the 'value-free' objective of health promotion includes providing **appropriate** knowledge of how to be 'healthy', the 'experts' who officially deliver such knowledge do so as employees of the same 'moral state' that condemns the patients they treat, which suggests that the objective is institutionally unobtainable. Superficially, the increased emphasis on empowerment practices acknowledges this basic contradiction. Supposedly enabling the patient/client to make 'comfortably and with confidence', choices between 'healthy' and 'unhealthy' practices, such empowerment could be little more than a more effective way of disciplining the patient, cajoled into believing she/he is exercising informed 'free' will, when in fact she/he is doing little more than showing the doctor that she/)he has learnt all she/he has been told.

Readers working in sexual healthcare will probably respond, but we are aware of all of this and our professional behaviour is informed accordingly. If so, my response is 'well some of you might be, but are you sure?' My lover died of an AIDS-related illness. Due to earlier unpleasant general healthcare encounters, one result of which was an HIV test made without his or my consent, he determined not to seek any medical care if he became ill. By the time he was taken into hospital, he was suffering from partial blindness and dementia, as a result of which he was simply categorised as 'in denial'. The nursing staff were 'well-intentioned' but offensive in their assumptions, allowing ministers and priests free access to patients too ill to refuse them. 'They are such a comfort' claimed one sister. 'Not if you are an atheist' I replied. Physically barring the way to one priest and having to shout to stop him 'don't you ever try and enter this room again', he replied 'God bless you my son'. Ultimately 'making sense of sexuality' is recognising that even in one such brief phrase, encountered in one brief, bleak interaction, sexualities are forged out of discourses laced with controlling power.

Notes

[1] Coxon, T and Carbello, M (1989): 'On the one hand 'community' is a device that homogenises, suppresses internal differences, creates exclusionary boundaries and functions as a dynamo of separatism. In practice, however, 'community' is a site of resis-

tances, of strategic essentialism and strategic difference. But 'community' at any time is less than 'stable' and all the more so for the stigmatised 'gay and lesbian constituency' (Woodhead, 1995).

2   In the Netherlands, police retreated from gay bathhouses where owners agreed to promote safe sex information and practices. French survey showed that safe sex promotion was less likely in establishments where provisions for sexual encounters were made a paradox explained in terms of 'men come here to relax'.

Bibliography

Amis M (1985) Making sense of AIDS. *The Observer*, 23rd June: 22

Aristotle (1972) *Politics*. Penguin, Harmondsworth

Bauman Z (1988) Sociology and postmodernity. *Sociol Rev* **36**: 796–813, 807

Bayer R (1989) *Private Acts, Social Consequences: AIDS and the Politics of Public Health*. Free Press, New York: 26–7

Bell D, Valentine G, eds. (1995) *Mapping Desire*. Routledge, London

Bloor M (1995) *The Sociology of HIV Transmission*. Sage, London

Bochow M (1990) AIDS and gay men: Individual strategies and collective coping. *Eur Sociol Rev* **6**(2): 124–8

Brogan DW (1960) *Citizenship Today*. University of Carolina Press, Chapel Hill

Coxon T (1988) The numbers game — gay lifestyles: epidemiology of AIDS and social science. In: Aggleton P, Homans H, eds. *Social Aspects of AIDS*. Falmer, London

Coxon T, Carbello M (1989) Editorial review: research on AIDS: behavioural perspectives. *AIDS* **3**: 191–7

Davies C (1975) *Permissive Britain: Social Change in the Sixties and Seventies*. Pitman, London

Day S (1988) Prostitute women and AIDS: Anthropology. *AIDS* **2**: 421–8

Department of Health (1991) *Citizens Charter; Raising the Standard*. Cmnd. 1599, July. HMSO, London

Dreuilhe E (1987) *Mortal Embrace: Living with AIDS*. Faber and Faber, London: 1

Evans DT (1989/90) Section 28: law, myth and paradox. Crit Social Policy **27**: 73–95

Evans DT (1993) *Sexual Citizenship: The Material Construction of Sexualities*. Routledge, London

Featherstone M (1988) Body and consumer culture. *Theory Cult Soc* **1**:18–33; **2**: 19

Foucault M (1981) *The History of Sexuality Volume One: An Introduction*. Penguin, Harmondsworth

Foucault M, Sennett R (1981) Sexuality and solitude, *Humanit Rev* **1**(3): 21

Freud S (1977: 1905) Three essays on the theory of sexuality. In: Richards A, ed. *Sigmund Freud: Volume 7: On Sexuality*. Penguin, Harmondsworth

Gagnon JH (1967) Sexuality and sexual learning in the child. In: Gagnon JS, Simon WH, eds. Sexual Deviance. Harper and Row, London

Gagnon JH, Simon WS (1967) *Sexual Deviance*. Harper and Row, London:

Gagnon JH, Simon WS (1968) The social meaning of prison homosexuality. *Fed Prob* **32**: 23–9

Gagnon JH, Simon WS (1969) Psychosexual development. *Transact* March: 9–17

Gagnon JH, Simon WS (1970) *The Sexual Scene*. Aldine, Chicago

Gagnon JH, Simon WS (1973) *Sexual Conduct: The Social Sources of Human Sexuality*. Aldine, Chicago

Gagnon JH, Simon WS (1986) Sexual scripts: permanence and change. *Arch Sex Behav* April: 97–121

Greer G (1984) *Sex and Destiny: The Politics of Human Fertility*. Secker and Warburg, London:

van Griensven GJP (1987) Risk factors and prevalence of HIV antibodies in homosexual men in the Netherlands. *Am J Epidemiol* **125**(6): 41–2

Hall S (1979) Reformism and the legislation of consent. In: National Deviancy Conference, Editorial. *Permissiveness and Control*. Macmillan, London

Hamer D, *et al* (1993) A linkage between DNA markers on the X chromasome and male sexual orientation. *Science* **261**: 321–7

Harris CC (1970) *The Sociology of the Family*. Macmillan, London

Hawkes G (1996) *The Sociology of Sex and Sexuality*. Open University Press, Milton Keynes

Heath S (1982) *The Sexual Fix*. Macmillan, London

Hobsbawm E (1981) The formal march of labour halted? In: Jacques M, Mulhern F, eds. *Observations on the Debate*. New Left Books, London

Kinsey KC, Pomeroy WB, Martin CE (1948) *Sexual Behaviour in the Human Male*. W B Saunders, Philadelphia

Kinsey KC, Gebhard P, Pomeroy WB, Martin CE (1953) *Sexual Behaviour in the Human Female*. W B Saunders, Philadelphia

Lees S (1993) *Sugar and Spice*. Penguin, Harmondsworth

Mac an Ghaill (1994) *The Making of Men*. Open University Press, Milton Keynes

McCaffrey J (1972) *The Homosexual Dialectic*. Prentice-Hall, New Jersey

McIntosh M (1968) The homosexual role. *Soc Prob* **16**(2): 182–92

McIntosh M (1978) Who needs prostitutes: The ideology of male sex needs and female attractiveness. In: Smart C, Smart B, eds. *Women, Sexuality and Social Control*. Routledge and Kegan Paul, London

McKeganey N, Barnard M (1996) *Sex Work on the Streets*. Open University Press, Milton Keynes

Marquet J, Hubert M, van Campenhoudt L (1996) Public awareness: discrimination and the effects of mistrust. In: Fitsimmons D, Hardy V, Tolley K, eds. *The Economic and Social Impact of AIDS in Europe*. Cassell: London: 219–33

Marshall TH (1950) *Citizenship and Social Class and Other Essays*. Cambridge University Press, Cambridge

Mead M (1935) *Sex and Temprament in Three Primitive Societies*. Gollancz, London

Mort F (1980) Sexuality, regulation and contestation. In: Gay Left Collective, ed. *Homosexuality, Power and Politics*. Allison and Busby, London

Plummer K (1975) *Sexual Stigma: An Interactionist Account*. Routledge and Kegan Paul, London

Pollak M (1988) *Les homosexuels et la sida. Sociologie d'une épidémie*. Anne-Marie Métailié, Paris

Pollak M (1992) *AIDS: A Problem for Sociological Research*. Sage, London

Pollak M (1994) *The Second Plague of Europe: AIDS Prevention and Sexual Transmission among men in Western Europe*. Harrington Park Press: Haworth NY: 63

Pollack M, Schiltz M-A (1991) *A Six Year Study of Bisexual and Gay Men with AIDS*. CNS-MIRE, Paris

Prieur A (1990) Norwegian gay men: reasons for continued practice of unsafe sex. *AIDS Educ Prev* **2**(2): 109–15

Rawls J (1972) *A Theory of Justice*. Oxford University Press: Oxford

Rawls J (1987) The basic liberties and their priority. In: McMurrin S, ed. *Liberty, Equality and Law*. University of Utah Press and Cambridge University Press, Salt Lake City and Cambridge

Rühmann F (1985) *AIDS: Eine Krankheit und ihre Folger*. Qumran, Frankfurt

Section 28 Local Government Act (England and Wales) (1988). *Scottish Current Law Statutes 1989*

Seidman S (1989) Transfiguring sexual identity. AIDS and the contemporary construction of homosexuality. *Theory Cult Soc* **6**: 293–315

Siegel K, Bauman LJ (1986) Methodological issues in AIDS related research. In: Feldman DA, Johnson TM, eds. *The Social Dimensions of AIDS*. Praeger, New York

Vance C (1988) Social construction theory: problems in the history of sexuality. In: Altman D *et al*, eds. *Homosexuality? Which Homosexuality?* Gay Men's Press, London and Amsterdam

Watney S (1988) AIDS, "moral panic" theory and homophobia. In: Aggleton, P, Homans H, eds. *Social Aspects of AIDS*. Falmer, London

Weber M (1967) Class, status and party. In: Gerth HH, Mills CW eds. *From Max Weber*. Routledge and Kegan Paul, London: 181

Weeks J (1995) History, desire and identities. In: Parker RG, Gagnon JH eds. *Conceiving Sexuality: Approaches to Sexuality in the Postmodern World*. Routledge, London

Wolfenden Report (1957) *The Report of the Committee on Homosexual Offences and Prostitution*. Cmnd. 247. HMSO, London

Woodhead D (1995) Surveillant gays: HIV space and the constitution of identities. In: Bell D, Valentine G, eds. *Mapping Desire*. Routledge, London

Zich J, Temoshok L (1986) Applied methodology: a primer of pitfalls and opportunities in AIDS research. In: Feldman DA, Johnson TM, eds. *The Social Dimensions of AIDS*. Praeger, New York

2
Multiple positions: a philosophical approach to sexual health

Robert-Gareth Hill

> 'Healthy Sexuality' is a chameleon concept. On the one hand, it seems that nothing could be easier to understand, or that there is nothing to be understood. The concept of 'healthy sexuality' does not arise naturally in our biographies. We learn at our mothers' knees (or nearby) what is right, decent, proper sexual behaviour. She uses the language of morals, not the language of health. So there is nothing to be understood. When health is mentioned at all, we are told to keep our body-parts clean and we learn about venereal disease. So 'healthy sexuality' is easily understood in terms of soap and penicillin.
>
> (Soble, 1987)

Introduction

Philosophy and sex or the conjoining of thought and feeling/action have tended to be separated within the western philosophical tradition (Marcuse, 1955). In part, this is due to Descartes strict delineation between the thinking subject and the experiencing body, but also because of the Judaeo-Christian divide between activities of the flesh and activities of the spirit, 'For the flesh lusteth against the spirit and the spirit against the flesh: and these are contrary the one to the other. So that ye cannot do the things that ye would' (Galatians 5.17). Such rigid demarcation lines seem to be breaking down, partly as a result of increasing western secularisation, partly through the philosophical advances made by Freud and psychoanalysis, and partly through a European tradition of philosophy that has always placed a greater emphasis on questions surrounding the body and its activities. Yet it is not these factors alone which have caused the increase in interest in the issue of sexual health. As Kolodny (1987) states, 'What constitutes a healthy sexuality has changed considerably over the past hundred years, indicating both a change in beliefs informed by advancing scientific knowledge and a reconsideration of 'health' and 'normality' in light of changing cultural mores and practices'. One only has to consider examples, such as the change in the conception of masturbation, from the Enlightenment (Hare, 1962; Tarczylo, 1987) to the current celebratory approach (Dodson, 1996), or the gradual abandonment of the disease concept of homosexuality to its current standing as a way of being in the world (Hansen, 1992). Thus, we can recognise that sexual health is both a historically and contemporaneously constructed concept.

A second reason for our interest in sexual health is the emergence of new technologies, technologies that in a purely functional sense can already supplant the sexual act (Beller, 1987). As a result, a new set of questions on the borderland between ethics and law have arisen and, while such interest does not neglect the long-standing interest shown by theologians and educators in questions surrounding sexuality, it does relocate it in a set of new moral arguments and cultural determinants. More than ever before we need to know what it is that sexual health stands for: moral fortitude, social well-being, the absence of disease, the maximisation of physical and mental pleasure, the medicalisation of instinctual activities, nothing? Whatever it turns out to be, our modern world consciousness suggests that it will not simply be a product of our psychological, sociological and biological selves, but that it will have emerged and been sanctioned from within the cultural context in which we live. If there is no other reason why sexual health must be questioned, it is because its area is wide and boundaries unclear. This does, however, open us up to a peculiar problem. Heidegger (1958) in his discussion on the nature of philosophy put the problem thus:

> *With this question we are touching on a theme which is very broad, that is, widespread. Because the theme is broad, it is indefinite. Because it is indefinite, we can treat the theme from the most varied points of view. Thereby we shall always hit upon something that is valid. But because, in the treatment of this extensive theme, all possible opinions intermingle, we are in danger of having our discussion lack proper cohesion.*

Such a passage serves as a useful reminder that it is not only the subject matter of sexual health, but our method of inquiry 'philosophy' that is problematic. Why take a philosophical perspective at all? What is it about philosophy that is important when considering the nature of sexual health?

Why philosophy?

Philosophy ('philosophia', literally the love of wisdom) is often held up as an example of abstruse thought, of concern to only a limited number of individuals and irrelevant to the concerns of everyday life. As Wittgenstein said:

> *What is the use of studying philosophy if all that it does for you is to enable you to talk with some plausibility about some abstruse questions of logic, etc, and if it does not improve your thinking about the important questions of everyday life ..?*

(Flew, 1979)

Philosophy can be both esoteric and inaccessible, although this is not always the case, nor was this the original impulse to philosophise:

> *This sense of wonder is the mark of the philosopher. Philosophy has no other origin and he was a good genealogist who made Iris (philosophy) the daughter of Thaumas (wonder). (Theatetus, 155,d)*

(Cornford, 1979)

Philosophy emerged from a desire to understand the nature of the universe in a rational way. Understood thus, it is undoubtedly a complex activity, dealing as it does with questions concerning the nature of knowledge, the nature of being and issues concerning freedom, immortality and good versus evil. Yet, can we be any more precise? Flew (1979) reports that G E Moore when asked 'What is this subject, this discipline?' gestured towards his bookshelves and said 'It is what all those are about.' What is intriguing about Moore's ostensible definition is that we do not know the nature of the books on his bookshelf towards which he gestured. It is this which raises an interesting question in philosophy, namely whether philosophy is characterised by its treatment of a philosophical subject matter, or whether philosophy is an approach or set of skills applicable to any and all subjects. If Moore's bookcase contained books on philosophical subjects (however they may have come to be defined) we can say what philosophy is by simply cataloguing what philosophers have talked and written about. If, on the other hand, Moore's bookshelf contained historical books, works of fiction and so forth, we need to discover what it is that connects them to the term 'philosophical'. One answer could be that such books are philosophical by dint of a certain conceptual approach. Thus it is possible that Moore's bookshelves contained a wide variety of books — books on philosophical subjects and books with a philosophical approach, some of the former containing both elements. If any books remained, we could always suggest, rather unsatisfactorily, that philosophy is foundational in respect of culture and that whatever the nature of the remaining books, philosophy will have had a part to play in their formation. Thus philosophy could be said to come into being, either by the nature of the questions that it asks, (what is knowledge, how do we know right from wrong, etc.) or through a distinct conceptual approach to such questions.

This chapter adopts a conceptual approach to a non-philosophical subject — sexual health; an approach that is increasingly being recognised as important:

> ... when clinicians discuss sexual matters with their patients, they attempt to do so in a manner that draws appropriately on their scientific knowledge and therapeutic training. The point to be taken is that when sexual events conspire to force patients to engage their clinicians in discussions of sexual matters, the discussion necessarily evokes philosophies of sex, not because clinicians act in an unscientific or non-therapeutic manner, but rather because both science and therapy presuppose normative and philosophical commitments.
>
> (Baker, 1987)

The remainder of this chapter examines the nature of sexual health from just such normative and philosophical commitments, by analysing ways that the term 'sexual health' can be constructed. The final section of the chapter briefly suggests some of the benefits of employing a philosophical approach to issues of sexual health.

Before turning to these tasks, it is worth pointing out the perspective that has been adopted in this chapter when considering sexual health. There is a tradition of philosophy in which language is seen as the solution to the philosophical puzzle (Hampshire, 1967). From such a perspective, an analysis of the constituent parts of a term is a preparatory activity in identifying the meaning behind the whole term. While there are undoubtedly situations where such an approach is worthwhile, the author does not believe this holds in the case of sexual health. The likelihood of sexual health taking on an invariant character when dissected into the constituent parts, **sexual** and **health** is minimal, a fact Soble (1987) reminds us of when talking about sexual health as a chameleon concept. Two passages highlight the potential difficulties:

> 'Seriously, it is not so easy to decide what is covered by the concept 'sexual'. Perhaps the only suitable definition would be 'everything that is related to the distinction between the two sexes'. But you will regard that as colourless and too comprehensive. If you take the fact of the sexual act as the central point, you will perhaps define as sexual everything which, with a view to obtaining pleasure, is concerned with the body, and in particular with the sexual organs of someone of the opposite sex, and which in the last resort aims at the union of the genitals and the performance of the

sexual act. But if so you will really not be very far from the equation of what is sexual with what is improper, and childbirth will really not be anything sexual. If, on the other hand, you take the reproductive function as the nucleus of sexuality, you risk excluding a whole number of things which are not aimed at reproduction but which are certainly sexual, such as masturbation and perhaps even kissing. But we are already prepared to find that attempts at a definition always lead to difficulties; so let us renounce the idea of doing better in this particular case. We may suspect that in the course of the development of the concept 'sexual' something has happened which has resulted in what Silberer has aptly called an 'error of superimposition'.

(Freud, 1981)

'. . . health, unlike traffic, cannot be defined, or, rather, is the setting of a continual struggle over definition, a struggle arising from the need to gain control over the realm of the transhistorical, ie. nature, or the body.'

(Kovel, 1982)

If we accept that 'errors of superimposition' (the idea that one is looking at one thing only) can and do occur, then not only will an analysis of the constituent parts of the term 'sexual health' be difficult, but also unlikely to help us in our examination of sexual health. Thus, in this chapter, sexual health will be treated as a potentially meaningful term, but one whose coherence and subsequent utility will have to judged on the particular constructs underlying the term and not on the constituent parts of the term itself. Philosophically, the approach adopted owes a great deal to the ideas expressed by Rorty in *Philosophy and the Mirror of Nature* (1979). From Rorty's perspective, there is no privileged standpoint by which we can judge competing claims to knowledge, and we should embrace philosophy for the clarity it brings to the questions it asks. Philosophy understood in this way is more a case of an edifying conversation than an objective epistemology.

A historical and contemporary overview of sexual health

It is important to remind ourselves that the world in which sexual health figures as a discourse is relatively new. Indeed, the OED points out that 'sexuality' as a term only appeared in 1800, tying it, as Caplan (1987) points out, to modern society. This does not mean that considerations over morality or immorality in terms of relationships between individuals is new, nor to suggest that people have only recently become aware of the risks connected to the sexual act, to procreation and the fleeting encounter. Indeed, it is only recently that venereal disease has become a controllable sexual risk and the western medical approach to childbirth a minimal risk to woman's mortality (Lane, 1995). Rather, it is that our discourse about sexual health is a modern phenomenon and it is with some justice that, prior to this, we were caught in the jaws of our own reproductive abilities.

There are four main bodies of work that have helped to stimulate our interest in sexual health. Firstly, there is the tradition of psychoanalysis inaugurated by Freud and taken into the social realm through the healthy 'sex economy' of Wilhelm Reich. Although Freud and Reich are not 'philosophers' in the restricted academic sense of the term, there is little doubt that their work, while tied to empirical means of investigation, emerged from a set of philosophical assumptions. Freud distinguished philosophy and science in the following manner:

> 'Philosophy is not opposed to science, it behaves like a science and works in part by the same methods; it departs from it, however, by clinging to the illusion of being able to present a picture of the universe which is without gaps and is coherent, though one which is bound to collapse with every fresh advance in our knowledge. It goes astray in its method by over-estimating the epistemological value of our logical operations and by accepting other sources of knowledge such as intuition'.

(Freud, 1973)

The second body of work emerged out of the work of continental philosophy, phenomenology, existentialism and postmodernism. Of particular importance is the work of Sartre (1991), Merleau-Ponty (1962) and feminist philosophers, such as Simone de Beauvoir (1953) and Luce Irigray (1992). Such writers recognised the importance of 'the body' and saw it less as an empty vessel controlled by consciousness, and more as a state of being, creating and in turn created, both by desire and the Other. 'The first apprehension of the Other's sexuality in so far as it is lived and suffered can be only desire; it is by desiring the Other (or by discovering myself as incapable of desiring him) or by apprehending his desire for me that I discover his being-sexed. Desire reveals to me simultaneously my being-sexed and his being-sexed, my body as sex and his body' (Sartre, 1991). Foucault, similarly, in his wide-ranging work points out the relative, socially meaningful and constructed nature of the conceptual world we inhabit, madness becoming defined not through psychiatry, but psychiatry through the labelling of the mad, and sexuality 'an especially dense transfer point for relations of power . . . endowed with the greatest instrumentality: useful for the greatest numbers of manoeuvres and capable of serving as a point of support, as a linchpin, for the most varied strategies' (Foucault, 1981).

The third body of work of importance is the literature on the cultural construction of sexuality. There is now an established body of work that shows how conceptions of sexuality are created and defined from the cultural milieu within which we live (Caplan, 1987), work which has been examined elsewhere in this book. For the purposes of this chapter, it is sufficient to remind ourselves that sexuality is not simply a historically constructed, but also a culturally defined conception. In the global village, conceptions of sexuality will inevitably be multifaceted and constructed not simply from tradition and culture, but also from our ever expanding knowledge and information networks, networks which in a very real sense are in perpetual transition. Butler (1993) points out that queer theory/politics:

> 'still . . . pose[s] the question of 'identity', but no longer as a pre-established position or a uniform entity; rather, as part of a dynamic map of power in which identities are constituted and/or erased, deployed and/or paralysed.'

Finally, there is a body of work concerned with sexual health undertaken and, some like Illich (1976) would argue, created by physicians, psychiatrists, prison psychologists and other health professionals who are in contact with individuals who suffer a variety of disorders of self and other problems, such as gender identity. Much of this work is therapeutic in intent and follows a fairly clearly defined conception of sexual normality and, therefore, health. A related body of work concerns itself with reproductive technologies, fuelled partly by our increasing technological expertise and partly by our changing cultural mores. It is these two areas of applied sexual health that are most likely to impinge upon health professionals in the course of their working lives.

The concept of sexual health

What sexual health means is not obvious. Some writers identify it in terms of a set of healthy moral practices, others pinpoint it negatively as the absence of disease, others as the absence of certain perversions, still others see it as an entirely relative concept dependent upon the reasons or justifications of the persons involved. Conceptually, there is no one 'sexual health' and it is in this context that philosophy can help outline the range of meanings attached to the term. However, although there is no one 'sexual health', there are a number of ways of considering it. Thus one can conceptualise sexual health as:

(i) an instinctual drive that, left unfettered, will automatically result in the development of a healthy sexuality;

(ii) a practice that is a series of activities, which can be defined, usually on moral grounds, as sexually healthy as opposed to unhealthy;

(iii) a physical state; namely the condition in which a person minimally has an absence of disease, or is able to perform their sexual function adequately according to their current developmental stage;

(iv) a mental state, in which the individual conceives self or others in terms of sexual categories; and, finally,

(v) a state of social well-being in which the liberation of society is the mirror image of the liberation of the individual.

While these areas will be dealt with separately, it is important to note that these constructions could be superimposed upon each other in such a way that only one is visible, albeit in a distorted fashion. Thus while sexual health may be more or less coherent when examined from each perspective, we need to recognise that it is not fixed in any obvious sense and that each perspective is dependent upon its own often unstated evaluative assumptions.

(i) Sexual health as an instinctual drive

The importance of Freud (1961) and Reich (1993) for the history of sexuality cannot be underestimated, and both have done much to shape the ways in which we conceptualise the sexual. While both men held a number of more or less coherent theories in regard to sexuality (heterosexual genitility on the one hand and the instinctual object on the other), both have, at one point, viewed sexuality in terms of instinctual forces and suggested that, if individuals were able to live unfettered, then sexuality would instinctively develop in a certain direction or, as Soble (1987) states: 'if persons are free . . . their sexuality will develop according to the inner laws of the instinct itself, undistorted, unperverted, and healthy'. Both Freud and Reich identified the same restrictive structures: family, religion and education, although it would be fair to say that Reich believed in the possibility of overcoming such barriers in a more directly political and external way than Freud. However, while both men have differing conceptions in regard to what a healthy sexuality looks like, both develop their arguments inferentially. Thus they both believe that, because people who are not sexually healthy live restricted lives, the absence of such restriction will result in sexual health. This, as Soble (1987) points out, tells us only what healthy sexuality is intentionally, 'in another sense (extensionally), it doesn't tell us at all what items to assign to the two categories'. Thus psychoanalysis has left us with the enigma of trying to find individuals who have remained free to develop their sexuality without restriction and thereby instinctively. This type of argument has led to the anthropological gold rush in which the studied exception would actually become the universal or, as Soble (1987) puts it: 'Shiploads of European anthropologists thought the Holy Grail (of sexuality) would be found in the South Seas'. The exception, of course, has not been found and thus we remain unclear whether the instinctual drive theory leads us down the road of socio-biology (Symons, 1979) or down a more socially constructed lane. Thus the problem is one where we will have to wait for the conditions of life to change before the parameters of healthy sexuality can be defined. It is clear that such conditions are highly unlikely to emerge. Therefore, while the theory is open to empirical assessment, the conditions whereby we could do this remain improbable.

(ii) Sexual health as a set of practices

A second approach to sexual health is the idea that it consists of a set of practices centring around sex and which are defined in terms of health/illness on the basis of what we think of as acceptable. This at first sight seems reasonable, since the opposite of health need not be illness. Being unhealthy can be as much a moral designation as an 'objective' description of our mental or physical state. Thus sexual health viewed as a practice may be little more than the linguistic outcome of a set of moral or political axioms. Indeed, one has to ask who it is that is doing the defining? For instance, Suppe (1987) sees deviation as normality, 'Being different, deviation from some total conformity to some Victorian or any other sexual ideal is not abnormal; it is the very essence of normal sexuality'. Suppe is not making a moral point here, but one based on the evidence for the diversity of sexual acts. His argument is that psychiatry and medicine have misappropriated the sexual to the extent that, that which is not defined as a disorder can be construed in terms of health. Suppe states; 'Just as psychiatry and medicine invented The Homosexual, so too they have invented The Transvestite, The Pedophiliac, The Masochist, The Voyeur *et al*'. For Suppe, medicine and psychiatry have no authority over such areas and he argues that their current authority is 'unscientific and fraudulent'. Such a view has a long heritage, as the following passage from Plato (1951) indicates:

> '*A healthy body is admittedly different from a diseased body and unlike it . . . so the love which exists in a healthy body is different from the love which exists in a diseased body . . . It is the duty of a good practitioner to gratify the sound and healthy parts of the body and to thwart the unsound and diseased, and this is the*

> *business of what we call medicine, which is, in a word, the knowledge of the principles of love at work in the body in regard to repletion and evacuation. The most skilful doctor is the doctor who can distinguish between noble and base loves in this sphere, and the man who can cause a body to change the latter for the former, and can implant love in a body which lacks but needs it, and remove it where it already exists, will be a good practitioner.'*
>
> (Plato,1951)

While Plato formulated the 'noble doctor' who can distinguish between noble and base loves, we have a medicine transformed into a nominalistic psychiatry, one that constructs only to then diagnose elements of the construct. Suppe (1987) is clear that psychiatry and medicine have misappropriated notions of sexual abnormality and argues for a return to Kinsey:

> *'Viewed objectively, human sexual behaviour, in spite of its diversity, is more easily comprehended than most people, even scientists, previously have realised. The six types of sexual activity, masturbation, spontaneous nocturnal emissions, petting, heterosexual intercourse, homosexual contacts, and animal contacts, may seem to fall into categories that are as far apart as right and wrong, licit and illicit, normal and abnormal, acceptable and unacceptable in our social organisation. In actuality, they all prove to originate in the relatively simple mechanism which provide for erotic response when there are sufficient physical or psychic stimuli.*
>
> *To each individual, the significance of any particular type of sexual activity depends very largely upon his previous experience. Ultimately, certain activities may seem to him to be the only things that have value, that are right, that are socially acceptable; and all departures from his own particular patterns may seem to him to be enormous abnormalities . . . There is little evidence of the existence of such a thing as innate perversity, even among those individuals whose sexual activities society has been least inclined to accept. There is an abundance of evidence that most human sexual activities would become comprehensible to most individuals if they could know the background of each other's individual's behaviour.'*
>
> (Kinsey et al, 1948)

Suppe claims that if we do embrace this view, 'a medicine and psychiatry of sexuality will be quite unlike what we are accustomed to. But what authority they enjoy will then become as legitimate as their prior authority has been unscientific and fraudulent'. There is strength in Suppe's argument in that there appears little reason for 'disorders' as currently conceived to be categorised in such a simplistic culturally-determined fashion. Baker (1987), in an intriguing article, points out that many criticisms of anal intercourse rest on a view that it cannot be natural because it is non-procreative, he states 'But how does one know that nature intended no non-procreative acts? Perhaps nature intended some sexual activities to be non-procreative? Perhaps anal intercourse is a natural form of birth control?'

There are two further problems when considering sexual health as a set of practices. The first relates to the issue of the quantification of sexual functioning and the inevitably arbitrary line that is drawn between what is normal and abnormal. For instance, Kolodny (1987) asks how often, if at all, should vaginal orgasm occur for it to be considered healthy, or how long should a man have sexual intercourse before ejaculating? Clearly such speculations are not irrelevant if we want to state with any confidence the dividing line between health and illness. Secondly, one has to consider the exceptional case, the individual who chooses to be sexually abstinent. Is non-engagement in sexual acts indicative of a healthy sexuality or not? Here we are not talking about lack of desire, but rather volition. For instance, when this occurs in a religious community premised on the quest for a higher good, talk of sexual health appears irrelevant and dissipates as a meaningful category. Thus to equate sexual health with a set of practices appears to define it too narrowly. Indeed, to define sex as a set of practices is the real problem. The erotic, the fantasy, all would be disallowed if sex were to be conceived of as simply practice-based and it is the very essence of sexual arousal that such thoughts propel us towards the sexual act.

(iii) Sexual health as a physical state

> 'Sex, sex — what good does it do anyone to 'study' more and better orgasms, to open forbidden orifices, to experiment, to put himself into the satisfaction laboratory, the intensive care ward of 'fulfilment'. The body is a poor vessel for transcendance . . . Satiety, in life, is quick and inevitable. The return of anxiety, debts, bad luck, age, work, thought, interest in the passing scene, ambition, anger cannot be deferred by lovemaking. The consolations of sex are fixed and just what they have always been.'
>
> (Hardwick, 1978)

Sexual health conceived of in terms of a physical state can be formulated both positively and negatively, although the latter is probably more common in terms of self-designation. Negatively perceived, sexual health becomes an issue of illness either as a result of sexual acts resulting in diseases (sexually transmitted diseases), or because of non-sexual disabilities that affect the expression of sexuality or the performance of a sexual act. In the former case, there are the various types of venereal disease, passed on and caught through sexual acts, as well as diseases which, while not being restricted to the arena of sex, impact to a very large degree upon sexual acts because of the route of transmission, eg. HIV. In the second category there are all encompassing disabilities that impact upon sexual acts as well as those that are specifically associated with the sexual organs. There are also, of course, a wide range of disabilities, physical in origin, that impact upon sexual relationships in much the same way as they would impact upon other areas of life, eg. paralysis.

Conceiving sexual health in this negative way tells us very little about what it means to be sexually healthy, unless we simply mean by this the absence of physical disease. Yet such conceptions of health are no longer considered to be very useful, especially when we regard health in terms of complete physical, mental and social well-being. If health is no longer regarded as merely the absence of disease, what in physical terms would a healthy sexuality be? One approach would be to go along with the instinctual drive approach, but this would lead us into the cul-de-sac of trying to find examples of complete physical well-being isolated from the mental and social. Moreover, sexual health understood in a physical way raises interesting questions concerning the function of sex. If we are bodies engaging in acts without recourse to the mental, why do we do it? While Hardwick points out that our bodies are poor vessels for transcendence, what are we trying to transcend? Is the body able to transcend the body or is transcendence ultimately tied to the duality of the mind/body? Maybe the answer to a positive state of physical sexual health does then lie in the study of more and better orgasms, a calculus of sexual acts. The question that still needs to be asked is what a better orgasm conceived physically would be? If we want to isolate the physical from the mental then the best orgasm is one that fulfils its function. This looks like getting us remarkably close to an evolutionary theory of sexuality in the sense of a natural teleological view of sexual health. Sexual health thus becomes a natural readiness and ability to successfully procreate. Conceived of in this way, the young are adaptive sexual bodies and those unable to reproduce are bodies denied a state of sexual health. All of this assumes our natural function to be reproduction; if that is denied, what then? Clearly, there are problems associated with the physical conception of sexual health, particularly the fact that we exist in the world in more than just a physical sense. Sexuality honed to the most minute physiological detail neglects too much, as Merleau-Ponty (1962) states:

> '... the sexual life may, as in Casanova's case, for example, possess a kind of technical perfection corresponding to no particularly vigorous version of being in the world.'

Related to the idea of sexual health as a physical state is the idea of an aesthetics of sexual health (Harre, 1990). Through perceiving, can I perceive others as well as myself to be sexually healthy. People's explanations for engaging in unsafe sex practices results from the invisibility of signs of sexual disease on the other person. In Shilts' (1988) *And the Band Plays On*, Gaetan Dugas' patient, Zero, covered up his lesions, as it seemed they not only acted as obvious stigmata but also offended his own sense of his beautiful body:

> He didn't feel like he had cancer at all. That was what the doctor had said after cutting that bump from his face. Gaetan had wanted the small purplish spot removed to satisfy his vanity; the doctor had wanted it for a biopsy
>
> (Shilts, 1988)

Clearly, such an aesthetic is as much about the psychology of personal perception as it is to do with a pure aesthetic of the physical body. Whether there can, indeed, be an aesthetic of sexual health raises interesting questions concerning the relationship between the visible and the invisible, the social gesture and the sexual act.

(iv) Sexual health as a mental state

> 'Sex is defined by our ideas, not our bodies'
>
> (Solomon, 1987)

For much of the history of the western world, the notion that sexuality can be perceived as something which can be attributed to our mental state has not held strong currency. It is only with the decline in religious sensibility and the reformulation of sexuality into an issue of health as opposed to as issue of sin, that we have begun to view the possibility of there being a mental state that can be viewed as sexually healthy. In this modern sense, sexual health as a mental act is very much part of the relationship between our mental selves and those aspects of ours and others' world or behaviour which we identify as sexual. Clearly this opens up the possibility of everything being sexual and it is quite possible that everything has a sexual aspect for someone. Yet what situations are there in which our mental life could be described as sexually unhealthy? Put another way, in what context or with what type of mental act would a person believe him/herself to be sexually unhealthy?

From a religious or spiritual point of view, thoughts concerning sex may be considered unhealthy, but probably not as sexually unhealthy. While religions have certain sexual prohibitions, it is uncertain to what extent thoughts about sex are meaningfully categorised as sexually healthy. Thus, it may be that sexual health cannot be constructed in such a mentalistic fashion at all, since it assumes some normative mental content about sex that is either healthy or unhealthy. Such a course of action seems inappropriate unless we have recourse to the moral arguments, ie. thoughts about sex are wrong. However, as the author has indicated even where this holds, the designation would not be sexual ill health but immorality. There remains, however, sexual health as an absence of ideas and thoughts about sex that are experienced as disturbing to the individual. In one sense, this is the province of psychiatry and its nosology of sexual disorder. Understood thus, sexual health is not about the content of thought, but about whether such content causes distress or not to the individual. In this way, sexual health is a mental state in which we do not suffer psychological distress because of our 'sexual' thoughts, sexual ill health is what we do. The problem with this is that our thoughts about the sexual are unlikely to be understood negatively. In other words, our distress about the sexual content of our thoughts relates not to the sexual content alone, but to our beliefs about it, beliefs that will tend to be associated to other non-sexual beliefs. This suggests that we are on the wrong track and conceiving health in too mentalistic a fashion. Roger Scruton may be on the right track when he draws a distinction between health and happiness or between the condition of being an animal and the condition of being a human:

> *'Health is the state in which I flourish as an animal; happiness the state in which I flourish as a person. And it is an important feature of the ontological dependence of personhood — of its need to find embodiment in an animal life — that health is such an important precondition of happiness. But health is not everything; happiness requires that we flourish as rational beings. We must exercise our rational capacities successfully: we must be fulfilled as persons, through the decisions which guide our lives.'*
>
> (Scruton, 1986)

If sexual health is dependent upon our mental state, we need to be able to meaningfully categorise thoughts into health-related and illness-related. It is this that seems to defy us, unless we simply mean making judgments about activities. In its pure form, the question is what would it mean to have a sexually healthy consciousness in and of itself?

(v) Sexual health as societal well-being

The notion of sexual health as social well-being needs to be understood in terms that are wider than those of the individual (mentally or physically conceived), since well-being is predominantly defined through social categories, often political. Thus one's own sexual practices and manifestations are dependent upon the world in which they are undertaken. Sexual health here does not mean conformity, although that clearly is one possible way of seeing it if one equates social well-being with adjustment. Another way of talking about sexual health in this way is to recognise the interdependence of one's own sexuality with others.

In one sense the conditions laid down for the instinctual drive theory of sexual health require just such social well-being as the conditions for its emergence. Freud, despite what was said earlier concerning his instinct theory of sexuality, remains sceptical about the possibility of it emerging in our society. In *Civilisation and its Discontents* (1985), Freud argues that advanced society requires that our sexual energy is harnessed to the maintenance of the economic and cultural products of that society. Indeed, he seems to suggest that some degree of sexual dissatisfaction is necessary for the maintenance of higher civilised society. Such an argument was taken up and developed more fully by Herbert Marcuse in *Eros and Civilisation* (1955). For Marcuse, it is capitalist patriarchies that are antagonistic to sexual satisfaction. Thus sexual health emerges because the social conditions are right and if this is unlikely to occur in nation states where permissiveness is confused with freedom, it may be possible for such social conditions to occur in terms of intentional economic communities of acceptance and toleration.

The alternative view in terms of causation is that liberated sexuality will usher in a free and non-repressive society, a world reflected on by Winston Smith:

> 'You like doing this? I don't mean simply me: I mean the thing in itself?
>
> 'I adore it.'
>
> That was above all what he wanted to hear. Not merely the love of one person but the animal instinct, the simple undifferentiated desire: that was the force that would tear the Party to pieces.'

(Orwell, 1954)

Such instinctual desire could then be viewed as natural because:

> Natural sexual development is that development persons would undergo in the absence of social influences on their sexual

> *development; natural sexuality is that sexuality persons would exhibit were they never influenced by social factors*
>
> (Soble, 1987)

Yet viewing sexual health as either the cause or the outcome of a cherished social structure does not get us very far into the meaning of sexual health itself. Chiefly, this is because it suggests that if A exists then B follows and *vice versa*. But this tells us next to nothing about the core of a healthy sexuality, precisely because we have little sense of what it means to be free. Perceptions of heaven in which freedom rather than restraint are central, rarely focus on sexuality. Given our confusion over whether sexuality is a cause or function of freedom, we are naturally riven between the personal and the political.

Summary

In summary, some of the ways of approaching sexual health have been discussed in this chapter. As mentioned earlier, the demarcations do not necessarily reflect what any one individual means by sexual health. Nor is there likely to be something in the world we can label, isolate and categorise as sexual health, although such isolation can occur as a discipline, a creation, a result of a certain set of professional regulations, social customs and laws, evidenced by the existence of sexual counselling, family planning clinics, practical sexual health books, academic treatises and professional concern (Rose, 1989). To say that it is a creation not meant to denigrate it; indeed, the creation of a discipline of sexual health necessitates taking it seriously. Nor is it a case of giving up the ghost and locating its meaning in its products and external manifestations, as if that was the only place left to find it. Thus, what the author hopes to have shown are some of the ways of approaching the term and introduced some of the problems within each perspective. Of what utility are such speculations for health professionals?

Clinician philosophers?

Baker (1987), in a paper referred to earlier *The Clinician as Sexual Philosopher*, reminds us that, whether or not the clinician wants it, he or she invokes, when talking about sexual matters, certain 'normative and philosophical commitments':

> *'Nature knows no inconsistencies. The inconsistencies we find there are products of the interpretations we foist upon it when we reify our values as natural laws. In truth, however, neither nature,*

> *nor anatomy, nor any study of the prevalence of sexual practices can tell us whether it is proper to masturbate or to use contraceptives or to engage in anal intercourse. The answers to these questions, insofar as they have answers, can only be discovered in philosophical reflection.'*

Thus, those involved in issues of a sexual nature with their patients are involved with philosophy, whether they like it or not. While this may be absolutely correct, it paints too bleak a picture and does not do enough to articulate the potential benefits of addressing such issues from a philosophical perspective. This chapter proposes five reasons for adopting a philosophical approach to matters of sexual health.

Firstly, there is its stress on conceptual clarity, something which, while by no means being unique to philosophy, is of central importance. As the author hopes to have shown, what 'sexual health' means is not at all clear. Within each of the perspectives outlined is a whole array of suppositions, generally hidden but always waiting to come forth. Philosophy helps us to question our concepts and go beyond the intuitive. In this sense it helps us to remove bias and dogma from our thought and conversation. Left unquestioned, it is easy to assume that there is something called 'sexual health' waiting to be known. Sexual health is a multifaceted construct and one that can be approached in a number of different ways.

Secondly, there is the question of new technologies. Advances in science tend to create questions of an ethical nature. The philosophical treatment of ethics allows us to assess the relative merits of our decisions and to place them in a coherent framework of justifications. The literature and expertise in the area of medical ethics is growing and questions of ethics are rarely entirely separate from our activities and concerns.

Thirdly, health professionals increasingly work in environments in which they have to adjudicate between competing claims to knowledge. Often there are important epistemological questions at the basis of these debates, for example, transexualism and what it means to be a man or a woman. Such questions are not physiological, and philosophy reminds us that natural categories are not always meaningful categories. Philosophy in this sense helps us to recognise the assumptions on which many of our theoretical and active lives are based.

Fourthly, the work of particular philosophers can sometimes act as a useful starting point by which to understand particular issues of interest. For instance, Kierkegaard's (1980) conception of despair has been used to theoretically understand what may have been occurring in a case of child sexual abuse (Chung and Hill, 1993). The work of philosophers or clinicians adopting a philosophical perspective has the potential to be applied in a meaningful fashion to contemporary problems and issues. Moreover, increasingly, the divide between disciplines is breaking down, allowing for a more realistic and more complex understanding of the world.

Finally, much of philosophy is concerned with the questions of existence — 'Who am I? What does it mean to be human?' questions which health professionals are, in many respects, confronted with on a daily basis through their interactions with others. Health professionals are not unique but they are often in unique positions, confronted with unpalatable choices which cannot be abdicated. However we want to conceive of it, sexual health has a real effect upon people's lives and sense of identity.

Conclusion

This chapter has introduced the notion that sexual health is dependent both upon what is meant by the term and upon the current conception of what can be encompassed by the term. For example, sexual health may mean a set of practices that are defined as normal or at least non-pathological, as a mental state, physical state, state of social well-being and so forth. At the beginning of this chapter, it was suggested that to privilege one of these interpretations over and above any other would be misplaced. Sexual health does not exist as some Platonic form to which our interpretations only partially approximate. Rather, sexual health is a social construction and may well mean different things to the same person in different circumstances. There are a number of discrete ways of approaching the term, all of which hold some form of currency in the literature. These ways of approaching the concept are not meant to be comprehensive, nor does the author claim to have dealt with them in particular depth. However, he believes a philosophical approach, even when it does not provide any definitive answers, is extremely useful in defining questions. He stated earlier that his philosophical approach owes more to Rorty (1979) than anyone else and it seems appropriate to be clear about, not only the general epistemological perspective adopted, but also what this means in terms of the question of sexual health.

From his own perspective, he believes that sexual health is a term rich in confusion and thin in explanatory power. As an individual, he does not define himself or think of others in terms of sexual health or disease, although he admits to thinking of himself in terms of disease and others in a similar way, but the application of the adjective 'sexual' adds nothing. As a human being the state of health or disease is a manifestation of how any organism exists at a particular point. To think in terms of sexual health or disease is curious. At the most, this can associate particular states of illness with particular causative factors that may have resulted from a sexual act, but even here it seems more reasonable to think in terms of the act itself and not of the all encompassing notion of sexuality. Partially, this is because sexuality includes far more than any sexual act, while at the same time being an insufficient descriptor of being in the world. That there is a focus on issues surrounding sexual health is understood. However, such concerns emerge not from any natural impulse to conceive of ourselves in such a way, but simply through our ability to construct the world into more or less discrete segments. Whether the notion of sexual health has any mileage as an explanatory force remains to be seen. At the moment it would seem that we lack the conceptual schemes to progress very far. However, irrespective of whether or not such progression takes place, sexuality in all its myriad forms will remain our primary concern as human beings:

> 'Sexuality, it is said, is dramatic because we commit our whole personal life to it. But just why do we do this? Why is our body, for us, the mirror of our being, unless because it is a natural self, a current of given existence, with the result that we never know whether the forces which bear us on are its or ours — or with the result rather, that they are never entirely either its or ours. There is no outstripping of sexuality any more than there is any sexuality enclosed within itself. No one is saved and no one is totally lost.'
>
> (Merleau-Ponty, 1962)

Acknowledgements

I would like to thank Josephine Harrison, Ann McDonnell, Chris Porter and Diana Rose for their helpful comments on earlier drafts of this chapter.

References

Baker R (1987) The clinician as sexual philosopher. In: Shelp WE, ed. *Sexuality and Medicine, Volume II: Ethical Viewpoints in Transition*. D Reidel Publishing Company, Dordrecht: 87–111

Beauvoir S de (1953) *The Second Sex*. Capo, London

Beller FK (1987) A survey of human reproduction, infertility therapy, fertility control and ethical consequences. In: Shelp WE, ed. *Sexuality and Medicine, Volume I: Conceptual Roots*. D Reidel Publishing Company, Dordrecht: 87–111

Butler J (1993) *Bodies That Matter. On the Discursive Limits of Sex*. Routledge, New York and London:

Caplan P, ed. (1987) Introduction. In: *The Cultural Construction of Sexuality*. Tavistock, London

Chung MC, Hill RG (1993) On describing the psychological struggle of child sexual abuse victims through Kierkegaard's concept of self. *Child Psychiatry Hum Dev* **24**(2): 81–90

Cornford FM (1979) *Plato's Theory of Knowledge*. Routledge and Kegan Paul, London and Henley

Dodson B (1996 Revised) *Sex for One: The joy of self-loving*. TSP Paperbacks, London

Flew A (1979) *Philosophy: An introduction*. Teach Yourself Books, Hodder and Stoughton, London

Foucault M (1981) *The History of Sexuality, Volume 1: An introduction*. Penguin, Harmondsworth

Freud S (1961) *The Future of an Illusion*. Norton, New York

Freud S (1973) *New Introductory Lectures*. Penguin, Harmondsworth

Freud S (1981) *Introductory Lectures on Psychoanalysis*. Penguin, Harmondsworth

Freud S (1985) *Civilization, Society and Religion*. Penguin, Harmondsworth: 344–5

Hampshire S (1967) Are all philosophical questions of language? In: Rorty R ed. *The Linguistic Turn: Recent essays in philosophical method*. The University of Chicago Press, Chicago and London

Hansen B (1992) American physicians discovery of homosexuals, 1800–1900: A new diagnosis in a changing society. In: Rosenberg CE, Golden J, ed. *Framing Disease: Studies in Cultural History*. Rutgers University Press, New Brunswick, NJ: 104–33

Hardwick E (1978) Domestic matters. *Daedalus* **Winter**: 1–11

Hare EH (1962) Masturbatory insanity: the history of an idea. *J Ment Sci* **108**: 1–25

Harre R (1990) *Health as an Aesthetic Concept*. Spring, Cogito: 35–40

Heidegger M (1958) *What is Philosophy?* (Kluback W, Wilde JT translation). Twayne Publishers, New York

Illich I (1976) *Medical Nemesis*. Pantheon, New York

Irigray L (1992) *An Ethic of Sexual Difference*. Athlone Press, London

Kierkegaard S (1980) *The Sickness unto Death* (translated by Hong HV, Hong EH). Princeton University Press, Princeton, New Jersey

Kinsey A, Pomeroy W, Martin C (1948) *Sexual Behaviour in the Human Male*. WB Saunders, Philadelphia

Kolodny RC (1987) Medical and psychiatric perspectives on a healthy sexuality. In: Shelp WE ed. *Sexuality and Medicine, Volume I: Conceptual Roots*. D Reidel Publishing Company, Dordrecht: 3–16

Kovel J (1982) *The Age of Desire*. Pantheon, New York

Lane, K (1995) The medical model of the body as a site of risk: a case study of childbirth. In: Gabe J, ed. *Medicine, Health and Risk: Sociological Approaches*. Blackwell Publishers, Oxford

Marcuse H (1955) *Eros and Civilisation*. Beacon Books, Boston

Merleau-Ponty M (1962) *Phenomenology of Perception*. Translated by Smith C. Routledge and Kegan Paul, London

Orwell G (1954) *Nineteen Eighty-Four*. Penguin, Harmondsworth

Plato (1951) *The Symposium*. Translated by Hamilton W. Penguin Classics, Harmondsworth

Reich W (1993) *The Function of the Orgasm*. Translated by Carfagno VR. Souvenir Press, London

Rorty R (1979) *Philosophy and the Mirror of Nature*. Princeton University Press, Princeton

Rose N (1989) *Governing the Soul: The Shaping Of The Private Self*. Routledge, London

Sartre J-P (1991) *Being and Nothingness*. Translated by Barnes H. Routledge, London

Scruton R (1986) *Sexual Desire: A Philosophical Investigation*. Weidenfeld and Nicolson, London

Shilts R (1988) *And the Band Played On*. Viking, London

Soble A (1987) Philosophy, medicine and healthy sexuality. In: Shelp WE, ed. *Sexuality and Medicine, Volume I: Conceptual Roots*. D Reidel Publishing, Dordrecht: 111–39

Solomon RC (1987) Heterosex. In: Shelp WE, ed. *Sexuality and Medicine, Volume I: Conceptual Roots*. D Reidel Publishing, Dordrecht: 205–25

Suppe F (1987) Medical and psychiatric perspectives on human sexual behaviour. In: Shelp WE, ed. *Sexuality and Medicine, Volume I: Conceptual Roots*. D Reidel Publishing, Dordrecht: 3–16

Symons D (1979) *The Evolution of Human Sexuality*. Oxford University Press, Oxford and New York

Tarczylo T (1987) From lascivious erudition to the history of mentalities. In: Rousseau GS, Porter R, eds. *Sexual underworlds of the Enlightenment*. Manchester University Press, Manchester

3
Psychological perspectives on human sexuality

Ian Rivers

Introduction: sexuality in a sociocultural context

What is human sexuality? How can we define it? Many of us have a notion of what we mean when we say the word 'sexuality': for some it means nothing more than the physical act of sex; for others it is a descriptive term which relates to the sexual orientation or preference of an individual. In fact, it seems that those who research human sexuality have yet to agree unanimously upon a definition, and this has been due largely to their own, often idiosyncratic, usage of the term. In the opening paragraphs of their book *Human Sexuality in a World of Diversity*, Nevid et al (1995) illustrate the complexity of the term by drawing attention to the multifaceted nature of what it is to be a sexual being. They argue that human sexuality is not only about sexual behaviour, it is also defined by our gender and the way in which we act out our roles as men and women. Part of our sexuality comes from our ability to be aroused through fantasy and the eroticisation of objects, images and particular people. As they say, 'Our sexuality is an essential part of ourselves, whether or not we ever engage in sexual intercourse or sexual fantasy, or even if we lose sensation in our genitals because of injury.

Nevid et al (1995) go to great lengths to stress the fact that we live in a world of social, historical and cultural diversity, where the concepts of normality and abnormality with respect to human sexual behaviour are not as clearly delineated as we are often led to believe. Indeed, the evolution of medico-scientific disciplines, such as psychiatry and psychology, has resulted in the application of quite arbitrary benchmarks, which define those behaviours that are considered 'normal' and those that require some form of therapeutic or judicial intervention. For example, in the United Kingdom up until the 1930s, it was not unusual to find unmarried women, who had given birth to a child, confined indefinitely to a mental institution as a result of their perceived sexual misconduct; although the attitudes of the day ensured that no such fate befell unmarried fathers. It was only a decade later, in the United States, when Alfred Kinsey and his colleagues demonstrated that pre-martial sex was a relatively common experience among the under 25-year-olds (Kinsey *et al*, 1948).

Such examples make it clear that, in understanding human sexuality, we need to be sensitive to the changing pattern of our own society, and we must recognise that what is considered acceptable sexual behaviour today may have been considered unacceptable in the past or, by the same token, may be considered unacceptable at some point in the future. Furthermore, we should also recognise that the attitudes and beliefs of other cultures may not mirror our own and, as a result, we should guard against imposing a western pathology upon non-western cultures. Unfortunately, sensitivity towards cultural variations in the development and expression of human sexuality is relatively new to the disciplines of psychiatry and psychology. Historically, this has been the result of the predominance of Judaic-Christian philosophy and its determination of what constitutes 'normal' sexual behaviour. Consequently, as western nations expanded their empires and colonised 'new' territories, so too did the Christian church and, where conversion failed to change the sexual behaviours of many indigenous nations, psychiatry often stepped in to offer a convenient name or label for these wilful violations of social convention and canon law. For example, Williams (1992) demonstrates how turn-of-the-century anthropologists and ethnographers pathologised same-sex relationships among North American Indians without understanding their intrinsic value to the economic, social and spiritual life of the tribe. Even where researchers had taken the time to understand the traditional beliefs surrounding such relationships, Williams reports that many continued to use negative terminology, describing homosexuality as 'a social disorder' (Devereaux, 1937) or by pathologising an entire tribe: the anthropologist, Robert Lowie, once described the Crow as having, 'won the championship in unnatural practices' (Lowie, 1935).

In defence of these researchers, it is fair to say that the scientific study of sexuality was very much in its infancy at the time. It had been less than a century since Darwin had published *The Origin of Species* (1859) in which he set out his Theory of Natural Selection, challenging many traditionally held beliefs relating to the Creation. It had only been a matter of a few years since the first authoritative texts on the pathology of human sexuality had been published. Alfred Kinsey had yet to begin his research into the sexual behaviour of men and women in North America and, in the industrialised world, homosexuality remained an offence under the law. It is inevitable that such a backdrop had a profound effect upon the attitudes of many researchers, not to mention the publishability of their work.

Historical perspectives in the study of human sexuality

It was towards the end of the nineteenth century, when sexual repression was believed to be at its height (although the estimated number of prostitutes in London, for example, clearly indicates that this was not the case), that the scientific study of human sexuality began in earnest. In the United Kingdom between the years 1896 and 1910, Henry Havelock Ellis produced a series of volumes which he entitled *Studies in the Psychology of Sex*. Through his research, using case histories, medical records and anthropological evidence, Ellis argued that many of the sexual problems couples experienced were psychological rather than physical in origin (probably owing much to the fact that people could not discuss sexuality openly), and that it was entirely natural for women to have a healthy sex drive (previously it had been argued that women were born without any sexual drive whatsoever). He also argued that homosexuality was entirely natural and illustrative of the variability among normal, sexually healthy human beings. By comparison, Richard von Krafft-Ebing, a German psychiatrist, collected over 200 case studies demonstrating the pathological nature of human sexuality which he recounted in his book, *Psychopathia Sexualis* (1893). Although Krafft-Ebing's work has been described as both intolerant and lacking objectivity, it is worth noting that many of the disorders and dysfunctions he identified in the 1890s continue to feature in modern psychiatry. In addition, it was Krafft-Ebing who linked the term 'heterosexual' to reproductive sex and, by implication, to the concept of 'normality' whereas other eminent physicians and sexologists had made a distinct separation between sexual desire and procreation. For example, in 1892 in the *Chicago Medical Recorder*, James Kiernan had used the term 'heterosexual' to denote a particular form of sexual perversion. He had, in fact, argued that 'the hetero in these heterosexuals referred not to their interest in a different sex, but their desire for two difference sexes' (Katz, 1996). He believed that heterosexuals suffered from 'psychical hermaphroditism', and were to be considered more deviant than homosexuals who, he believed, were simply gender dysphoric (ie. they had the mental state of a member of the opposite sex).

Around the same time, in Vienna, Sigmund Freud was developing his theory of personality in which he argued that the principal forces behind motivation were sexual impulses or drives. Freud's theory rested on the belief that the underlying cause of several neuroses was the result of 'conflicts between the subject's sexual impulses and his [sic] resistance to sexuality' (Freud, 1935). Although Freud's work has been much criticised (particularly in relation to his advocacy of childhood sexuality), like Henry Havelock Ellis, he recognised that homosexuality was not an unnatural state: 'It can be traced back to the constitutional bisexuality of all human beings and to the after-effects of phallic primacy'. He argued further that his use of various descriptive terms such as 'polymorphously perverse' was, unlike many of his contemporaries, in no way meant to be judgmental. In his autobiographical study, he wrote: 'I was only using a terminology generally current; no moral judgment was implied by the phrase. Psychoanalysis has no concern whatever with such judgments of value'.

Perhaps the most important early contributor to the scientific study of sexuality was the German physician, Magnus Hirschfeld. Although Hirschfeld began his career in the field of public hygiene, his belief that the victimisation of homosexuals was unjustified resulted in his campaign for the reformation of the laws relating to homosexuality and bisexuality. In 1899, he founded the very first journal given over to the study of human sexuality, *The Journal of Intermediate Sex Stages*, and in 1913 he founded the Medical Society for Sexual Sciences. In 1918 he opened the Institute for Sexual Science in Berlin (later known as the Magnus Hirschfeld Foundation). Unlike Ellis, Krafft-Ebing and Freud, Hirschfeld employed scientific methodology to his studies of human sexuality. He was responsible for the very first survey of human sexual behaviour using a 130-item questionnaire which he distributed to 10 000 people; and he was the driving force behind the development of a number of centres which focused on the treatment of sexual problems. Although both Ellis and Freud had hinted at the innate nature of homosexuality, Hirschfeld argued that all sexuality (heterosexuality, homosexuality and bisexuality) was genetic in origin and not something that should be considered deviant or abnormal. Although much of his work, including the Magnus Hirschfeld Foundation, was destroyed by the Nazis in 1933, his application of a rigorous scientific methodology to the study of all aspects of human sexuality set a precedent for future researchers.

Some thirteen years after Hirschfeld's death, the zoologist Alfred Kinsey, together with two colleagues (Wardell Pomeroy and Clyde Martin), published their investigation into the sexual behaviour of American men (Kinsey *et al*, 1948). Five years later, with another colleague, Paul Gebhard, Kinsey, Pomeroy and Martin published a second comparative study focusing upon the sexual behaviour of American women (Kinsey *et al*, 1953). Unlike Hirschfeld's earlier survey, Kinsey used a personal interview technique in gathering information about participants' sexual histories. Overall, both the Kinsey reports represented the results from in-depth interviews with 12 000 people living in the United States between the late 1930s and the early 1950s (Kinsey actually began his research in 1938 when he was asked to teach a course on marriage at Indiana University).

Although both the Kinsey reports represent a major advancement in our understanding of human sexual behaviour, at the time of their publication they were vilified in the press. In particular, scorn was poured on the second report *Sexual Behaviour in the Human Female* because it challenged the traditional myth that women were in some way less sexual than men. Indeed, Masters *et al* (1995) report that Kinsey was accused of being 'amoral, antifamily, and even tainted with communism' because he presented evidence which demonstrated that women were not born with a form of sexual anaesthesia which rendered them impervious to desire.

So, what exactly did Kinsey and his colleagues find in their research which so shocked the American press? Perhaps, their most startling revelation related to the incidence of post-pubescent homosexual sex in American men. No less than 37% of those men interviewed reported at least one homosexual experience resulting in orgasm after the onset of puberty. Other highly contentious results included the number of married men who reported being unfaithful to their spouses (40%); and the number of women who had tried masturbation (63%) (Masters, *et al*, 1995).

Although Kinsey and his colleagues had set a precedent for research into human sexuality, it was not until the mid-1960s that William Masters and Virginia Johnson published their own study relating to sexual arousal (Masters and Johnson, 1966). Masters and Johnson believed that, in addition to sexual behaviour, it was necessary to understand the physiological, psychological and sociological aspects of sexuality. They set up a laboratory-based investigation where they observed the sexual interactions of nearly 400 men and women, representing nearly 10 000 episodes of sexual activity. Like Kinsey, Masters and Johnson were criticised for the lack of morality in their research. However, this work led the way to a second, more important advancement in the study of human sexuality — the treatment of sexual problems. In their second volume, *Human Sexual Inadequacy*, Masters and Johnson (1970) described how they were able to help men and women with sexual problems in only two weeks with an 80% success rate. Previously, it had been the case that any form of sexual therapy had required lengthy treatment regimes without necessarily yielding a high rate of success. Within a few short years a revolution in sexual therapy took place: clinics and centres were opened across the United States, and sex and sexuality became issues which could be discussed openly by the media.

Simultaneously, the gay rights movement was gaining momentum. Following the Stonewall Riots of 1969 (the result of protests against the raiding of a gay bar by police), campaigns to end lesbian and gay discrimination were launched across the country. In 1973, the

American Psychiatric Association declassified homosexuality as a mental disorder (the World Health Organization did not follow suit until 1992), although the classification ego-dystonic homosexuality continued to feature in American psychiatry until 1987 (American Psychiatric Association, 1987).

Despite the significant advances we have made this century in our understanding of human sexuality, there remains a great deal yet to discover. The advent of the AIDS epidemic has brought with it a re-evaluation of sexual behaviour among those communities most affected by it. Recently, there has been extensive research into the biological and genetic origins of sexual orientation, and the suggestion that male homosexuality may be linked to a particular area on the female chromosome (Xq28) (Hamer *et al*, 1993). Although we are now able to investigate theories relating to the genetic basis of human sexuality, it is worth remembering that such theories were first articulated by men such as Magnus Hirschfeld nearly a century ago.

Human sexuality and the normality/abnormality debate within psychology

Homosexuality/bisexuality

As previously stated, it was only a quarter of a century ago (in 1973) that the American Psychiatric Association removed homosexuality from their list of mental disorders. However, it was only in 1992 that the World Health Organization similarly removed homosexuality from their diagnostic manual, the *International Statistical Classification of Diseases and Related Health Problems*. Because such decisions were based upon social convention, this has allowed those who perceive homosexuality and bisexuality to be 'abnormal' to continue to offer cures and therapies which purport to alter a person's sexual orientation. Furthermore, because society continues to place a great deal of emphasis upon procreative (ie. heterosexual) sex, homosexual sex is often seen as recreative and, therefore, of less importance within relationships. This is clearly not the case as Flowers *et al* (1997) demonstrated: homosexual sex is an important feature in the definition and maintenance of a gay relationship, and the fact that the act of lovemaking does not result in the birth of a child is of little relevance to the longevity of that relationship.

Another recurrent theme, within the fields of psychiatry and psychology, has been whether or not much of the ongoing research relating to homosexuality/bisexuality illustrates the 'normal' development of lesbians, gay men and bisexual men and women. According to D'Augelli (1994), it is very difficult to get a sense of what it is like to grow up normally as a lesbian, gay man or bisexual man or woman because homosexuality is so stigmatised by society. Currently, much of the research examining homosexuality and bisexuality focuses upon the psychological consequences of living in a heterosexual world, and because of this emphasis upon the negative experiences of being lesbian, gay or bisexual, it seems very likely that researchers have unwittingly given ammunition to those who advocate the clinical abnormality and curability of homosexuality (Isay, 1989; Meyer-Bahlburg, 1990–91; Socarides, 1968). Despite such negativity, recent developments in the field of psychotherapy, particularly the evolution of 'affirmative' therapy, have offered an alternative perspective when examining the lives of lesbians, gay men and bisexual men and women.

As its name implies, the very existence of an alternative and 'affirmative' psychotherapeutic discipline suggests that other forms of therapy portray an individual's sexual orientation as a significant factor (if not the root cause) of psychological disturbance. 'Affirmative' therapy works on two very basic principles:

(i) that being lesbian, gay or bisexual is a natural, healthy alternative to heterosexuality, and the role of 'affirmative' therapy is to work towards the self-actualisation of the individual rather than uncovering their pathology;

(ii) that being lesbian, gay or bisexual is not the cause of an individual's distress, rather it is society's reaction to him/her which causes the distress.

This approach does have its critics from within lesbian and gay psychology, most notably Kitzinger and Perkins (1993) who have argued that providers of 'affirmative' therapy are, in fact, reinforcing the perception of illness and abnormality by using language such as 'homophobia', and through their willingness to 'cure' the ills lesbians, gay men and bisexual men and women face living in a heterosexual world. Although this is a negative and somewhat politicised view of 'affirmative' therapy, it is not without some foundation. As D'Augelli (1994) pointed out, within research, the social, medical and health sciences continue to pathologise every aspect of lesbian, gay and bisexual existence from adolescence to old age without establishing a concomitant body of research examining the pathology of anti-gay/lesbian/bisexual attitudes at a societal level

The sexual disorders

According to the American Psychiatric Association, there are three categories of sexual disorder; the paraphilias, the sexual dysfunctions and other sexual disorders which cannot be classified as either paraphilias or dysfunctions (a similar delineation is made by the World

Health Organization). Paraphilias are primarily disorders of arousal: they are characterised by the fact that a person with a paraphilia will be sexually aroused by objects or situations which do not conform to the so-called 'normal' arousal-activity patterns. On the other hand, sexual dysfunctions are not classified according to the atypicality of an individual's sexual behaviour, rather they represent interruptions in 'normal' sexual functioning. Clinical intervention and treatment of a sexual dysfunction occurs when one of the four stages of the sexual response cycle (appetitive, excitement, orgasm or resolution) is interrupted, and where such an interruption is persistent or recurrent. Currently, a range of therapies (behavioural, psychodynamic and humanistic) are available to individuals and couples who experience difficulties in their sex lives, and many of these therapies were developed as a direct result of Masters and Johnson's research in the late 1960s and early 1970s.

It is arguable that, unlike the sexual dysfunctions, the paraphilias represent an area of human sexuality where there has been little development in our understanding since the publication of Krafft-Ebing's volume of case studies in 1893.

Rather than being defined solely as a range of mental disorders which either cause distress to the individual or to those closest to them, they represent not only medical judgments about the sexuality of an individual, but also a wide range of cultural, social and moral judgments of what constitutes 'normal' sexual behaviour.

The paraphilias include behaviours such as sexual fetishes and transvestic fetishes, voyeurism, frotteurism, exhibitionism, sexual masochism, sexual sadism and paedophilia. Some paraphilias only occur during times of stress, or at times when a person is unable to maintain a sexual relationship without resorting to a fantasy or stimulus. The individual's use of imagery is an important factor in the determination of whether or not they suffer from a paraphilia. However, as most people use some form of imagery or fantasy to elicit sexual arousal (especially during masturbation), it can be difficult to separate the 'normal' from the 'abnormal'. In psychiatric terms, the use of a particular fantasy or stimulus to aid arousal becomes a paraphilia when it causes persistent distress to the individual (for six months or more), or when the individual's behaviour causes distress to another (usually an unwilling participant). Yet, it cannot be classified as a paraphilia *per se* when the fantasy or stimulus does not cause distress, regardless of its atypicality. Generally, such definitions are reflected in the law and, when they are brought to trial, behaviours, such as voyeurism, frotteurism, exhibitionism and paedophilia can result in a custodial sentence for the offender (often with a psychiatric assessment or treatment order appended). But, it is also the case that the law in many countries does not recognise either masochism or sadism as alternative expressions of human sexuality, and even in cases where both partners have openly expressed their willingness to participate in sexual acts involving pain or humiliation, criminal convictions have followed. Thus, society's pre-judgment of what constitutes 'normal' sexual behaviour can, at times, be in direct opposition to both psychiatry and psychology, and this begs the question of 'who defines what is abnormal?'

Redefining 'normality': understanding cultural diversity

As the previous sections in this chapter have indicated, the scientific study of human sexuality is a relatively recent phenomenon and, as already indicated, although we have made significant advances in our understanding of all aspects of sexuality and sexual orientation, it would be presumptuous to assume that we have little left to learn. Because many of the ideas we have relating to the concept of abnormality with respect to human sexuality come from a western interpretation of what constitutes 'normal' sexual behaviour, this, as Williams (1992) demonstrates, has biased our view of sexual practices in other cultures. Indeed, it is only within the last few years that research in the field of cross-cultural psychology has gained momentum, and this has fortuitously coincided with the establishment of disciplines, such as psychological anthropology, which have given us a greater insight into the behaviours, traditions and beliefs of a variety of societies and cultures very different from our own. Indeed, it can be argued that nowhere has the establishment of these new disciplines had a greater effect than in our understanding of human sexuality.

Perhaps one of the best known studies, which challenges many of the ideas relating to 'normal' and 'abnormal' sexual behaviour, was conducted by Gilbert Herdt in New Guinea between 1974 and 1985. Herdt's research demonstrates how homosexuality and, more particularly, man-boy sexual relationships play an integral part in the development of young men from the Sambia tribe (see Herdt, 1981; 1984). The Sambia believe that while the ingestion of a mother's milk promotes the growth of a child, the ingestion of male semen by boys leads to their growth as hunters and warriors. From the age of seven, Sambian boys leave their mothers' side and go to live in the men's hut where they undergo a number of rituals which rid them of the pollution of living with women. For the remainder of their childhood and adolescence, the boys are required to fellate older men in the hut and, in turn, be fellated by younger boys when they have reached an appropriate age. As Herdt argues, both homosexual sex and man-boy relationships are intrinsic parts of the cycle of life for the Sambia: in order for a young boy to grow and become a strong warrior or hunter, they believe that he must ingest male semen. Thus, homosexuality in this context is not about the eroticisation of the penis, rather it is about the survival of the tribe, and its ability to produce strong men who can defend Sambian territory in times of warfare.

Although such beliefs may be difficult to accept for those of us brought up in a western tradition where there has always been a distinct separation between male and female, Herdt points out the Sambia believe that the first human beings were androgynous, and had both breasts and a penis. The folklore of the tribe tells how one of these androgynous beings became the first 'woman' when she fellated the other, the first 'man', causing her penis to disappear and her breasts to grow while, at the same time, causing the other's breasts to shrink. Although this tradition implies that a man who ingests the semen of another will become a woman, there is no evidence of gender confusion or dysphoria among the men of the tribe. In fact, it seems to have had the opposite effect, promoting masculinity through demonstrations of hunting skills and acts of bravery (Herdt, 1981).

Another example of cultural variations in the perception of sexuality and gender comes from Margaret Mead's study of the Tchambuli (also from New Guinea). Mead (1962) illustrated how many of the ideas we have relating to gender roles and the stereotypical behaviour of men and women in society do not transfer cross-culturally:

> 'The women go with shaved heads, unadorned, determinedly busy about their affairs. Adult males in Tchambuli are skittish (highly strung and fickle), wary of each other, interested in art, in the theatre, in a thousand petty bits of insult and gossip. The men wear lovely ornaments, they do the shopping, they carve and paint and dance. Men whose hair is long enough wear curls, and others make false curls out of rattan rings.'

Although much of Mead's work has been criticised for its reliance upon very subjective (ie. western) interpretations of male and female behaviour, her comments clearly show that some of the stereotypical attributions made about women in the west seem to be a feature of male behaviour among the Tchambuli. Could it be argued that the men and women of whom Mead wrote were suffering from some form of gender identity disorder? This seems very unlikely. However, the work of both Gilbert Herdt and Margaret Mead reinforce the belief that it is necessary for modern psychiatry and psychology to be sensitive to the cultural environment in which a person is raised. This does not relate solely to issues of sexuality and sexual orientation (although this is the primary focus of this chapter), it also relates to all aspects of psychiatric and psychological intervention.

Redefining 'abnormality': the anti-psychology approach

As far as possible, this chapter has presented different aspects of the normality/abnormality debate within the disciplines of psychiatry and psychology, with special reference to human sexuality. The concepts of 'normal' and 'abnormal' sexual behaviour are not fixed; they can vary across time and across cultures. However, it is not always the case that recognition of such variability is reflected by changes in clinical diagnosis and practice, and it may be worth considering why this is so. To a certain degree it can be argued that both psychiatry and psychology are victims of their own scientific approach to the study of mental illness. As illustrated in the titles of their diagnostic manuals, both the American Psychiatric Association (publishers of *The Diagnostic and Statistical Manual of Mental Disorders*) and the World Health Organization (publishers of *The International Statistical Classification of Diseases and Health-Related Problems*) base their judgments of what constitutes clinical 'abnormality' using a statistical 'norm' as their guide. This presents us with a number of problems in defining what exactly 'normality' is, especially when dealing with issues such as sexuality where previously there has been little discussion or research. For example, in 1995, in a letter to the editor of *The Psychologist* (the official organ of the British Psychological Society), one eminent British psychologist argued against the inclusion of an article on lesbian and gay relationships in a previous edition with the following statement:

> I object to the misleading use in a publication of a scientific society of the innocent-sounding word 'gay' when referring to what is the abnormal practice of anal intercourse between males. Secondly, I object to attempts to mislead readers about the epidemiological incidence and prevalence of male and female homosexuality which in statistical-mathematical terms is fortunately still tiny.
>
> Members should be aware that the terms 'normal', 'average', 'usual' or 'common' have basically a tight mathematical definition; they exclude scores, 'items', or people at a distance of two s[tandard] d[eviation]s from a 'mean'
>
> (Hamilton, 1995)

Although the anti-gay views expressed in this letter were condemned in subsequent letters to the editor, the inappropriate nature of a system of classification based solely upon mathematical principles is evident. Can we truly classify a person as 'normal' or 'abnormal' on the basis of whether or not they fall within or without two standard deviations from a calculated mean? The rigorous employment of such criteria would result not only in lesbians, gay men and bisexual men and women being labelled 'abnormal' once more, it would also result in the pathologisation of a number of other minority groups within society, such as infertile couples or disabled couples or, indeed, single men and women. Of course, the majority of practising psychiatrists and psychologists recognise that there are no hard and fast rules when dealing with human behaviour, and there is, increasingly, a recognition that variability exists not only between cultures, but also within them. Nevertheless, the usage of terms such as 'abnormal' when discussing aspects of human sexuality needs to be examined closely, and while not advocating the declassification of behaviours which cause distress to the individual or to others, it is clear that we need to be sensitive to environmental factors when assessing the normality or abnormality of a person's behavior.

Summary

The concepts of 'normality' and 'abnormality' with respect to human sexuality are not as clearly defined as they would first seem. Not only is there a great deal of variability within cultures in terms of sexual orientation and behaviour, variability also exists between cultures, and what we may consider 'normal' in our own culture can seem 'abnormal' or, perhaps, even 'perverse' in another and *vice versa*. Although both psychiatry and psychology have been slow to recognise the existence of such differences, the recent expansion in cross-cultural research offers us the opportunity to gain further insights into all aspects of human behaviour, taking account of cultural customs, beliefs and attitudes.

It is clear that the use of statistical classification systems for psychiatric disorders leaves a great deal to be desired, especially when addressing the issue of human sexuality. The fact that individual sexual behaviour does not conform to that of 95% of the population, does not necessarily mean that they are suffering from some form of psychiatric disorder. In many cases, it simply means that they have taken a different developmental trajectory in terms of sexual expression. The fact that alternative sexualities are often pathologised, or go unrecognised by society, is indicative of a need for a greater understanding and appreciation of human diversity.

References

American Psychiatric Association (1987) *The Diagnostic and Statistical Manual of Mental Disorders: Revised (DSM III-R)*. American Psychiatric Association, Washington, DC

Darwin C (1859) *The Origin of Species*. Murray, London

D'Augelli AR (1994) Lesbian and gay male development: steps towards an analysis of lesbian and gay men's lives. In: Greene B, Herek, GM eds. *Lesbian and Gay Psychology: Theory, Research and Clinical Applications*. Sage, Thousand Oaks, CA: 118–32

Devereaux G (1937) Institutionalized homosexuality of the Mohave Indians. *Hum Biol* **9**: 498–527

Flowers P, Smith JA, Sheeran P, Beail N (1997) Health and romance: understanding unprotected sex in relationships between gay men. *Br J Health Psychology* **2**: 73–86

Freud S (1935) *An Autobiographical Study*. Hogarth Press, London

Hamer D, Hu S, Magnuson VL, Hu N, Pattatucci AML (1993) A linkage between DNA markers on the X-Chromosome and male sexual orientation. *Science* **261**: 321–6

Hamilton V (1995) Are you normal? *The Psychologist* (Letters) **8**: 151

Herdt G (1981) *Guardian of the Flutes: Idioms of Masculinity*. McGraw Hill, New York

Herdt G, ed (1984) *Ritualized Homosexuality in Melanesia*. University of California Press, Berkeley, CA

Isay RA (1989) *Being Homosexual: Gay Men and Their Development*. Penguin, Harmondsworth

Katz JN (1996) *The Invention of Heterosexuality*. Plume, New York

Kinsey AC, Pomeroy WB, Martin CE (1948) *Sexual Behaviour in the Human Male*. WB Saunders, Philadelphia

Kinsey AC, Pomeroy WB, Martin CE, Gebhard PH (1953) *Sexual Behaviour in the Human Female*. WB Saunders, Philadelphia

Kitzinger C, Perkins R (1993) *Changing our Minds: Lesbian Feminism and Psychology*. Onlywomen Press, London

Krafft-Ebing R von (1893) *Psychopathia Sexualis, with Especial Reference to Contrary Sexual Instinct: A Medico-Legal Study*. FA Davis, Philadelphia

Lowie RH (1935) *The Crow Indians*. Farrar and Reinhardt, New York

Masters WH, Johnson VE (1966) *Human Sexual Response*. Little Brown, Boston

Masters WH, Johnson VE (1970) *Human Sexual Inadequacy*. Little Brown, Boston

Masters WH, Johnson VE, Kolodny RC (1995) *Human Sexuality*. Harper Collins, New York

Mead M (1962) *Male and Female*. Penguin, Harmondsworth

Meyer-Bahlburg HF (1990-91). Can homosexuality in adolescents be 'treated' by sex hormones? *J Child Adolesc Psychopharmacol* **1**: 231–5

Nevid JS, Fichner-Rathus L, Rathus SA (1995) *Human Sexuality in a World of Diversity*. Allyn and Bacon, Boston

Socarides C (1968) *The Overt Homosexual*. Grune and Stratton, New York

Williams WL (1992) *The Spirit and the Flesh: Sexual Diversity in American Indian Culture*. Beacon, Boston

World Health Organization (1992). *International Statistical Classification of Diseases and Related Health Problems: Tenth Edition* (ICD 10). WHO, Geneva

4
Sexuality and childbirth: towards a theory of female sexuality

Anna Sobolewski

The concept of sexuality in relation to childbirth can be seen as an anomaly. Pregnancy is usually the result of an act of sexual intercourse, yet the woman's sexuality thereafter tends to be forgotten. The literature predominantly discusses women's sexuality as a lack of getting back to normal (recommencing coitus) and ignores the psychological, physiological and hormonal effects of pregnancy, labour and the puerperium. These determine a slower resumption of the sex life which a couple may have experienced prior to childbirth. The adoption of a male model of sexuality as the norm has led to a medicalised view when discussing sexuality in childbirth. Perhaps this helps to desexualise the care given to a woman in pregnancy and childbirth, which is of a highly intimate nature. The attributes of 'woman' may be separated from the 'body 'so that doctors and midwives can distance themselves from their actions, making it difficult for the woman to gain help and support to express herself sexually during this time. Sexuality and motherhood are effectively split so that women cannot express their sexuality during their childbearing era (Ussher, 1993). It ignores the woman who may be coping with difficult feelings as a result of past sexual violence or abuse.

This chapter will review some of the research and theories, which have attempted to define female sexuality. It will be argued that an understanding of the historical, psychological, cultural, social and biological perspectives will enhance our current understanding of female sexuality. Then the literature relating to sexuality and childbirth will be examined, what makes childbirth sexual will be discussed and women who require special concern during pregnancy and childbirth will be highlighted. All women should be aware of the changes likely to occur to their sexuality or sexual responses during childbirth. This requires midwives and other childbirth educators to have an understanding of sexuality, and its specific aspects relating to childbirth, so that women will receive optimum care. It is not intended to analyse all the research individually but to give general comments about research into sexuality. The aim of the chapter is to aid practitioners in relating different perspectives of female sexuality to the concept of sexuality in pregnancy.

Towards a theory of female sexuality

Sex pervades our lives. It is difficult to define, but can be seen as an integral part of the human experience, for both males and females, a combination of sensual and erotic pleasure. We now consider a definition of female sexuality. Although the following is only one example, it can be used to indicate other aspects that need be considered when developing a theory. Since the definition of female sexuality lacks a clear conceptual framework, it is understandable that this lack of clarity continues when considering sexuality in relation to childbirth.

Bernhard (1995) states that 'female sexuality is a multidimensional, biopsychosocial phenomenon that consists of at least four components: sexual desire, sexual response, view of oneself as female, and presentation of oneself as woman'. Sexual desire is the urge for sexual activity and consists of how often a woman may want sex and whom she may prefer as a partner, eg. male, female or both. Sexual response refers to the physiological activities which are necessary for orgasm to occur. View of oneself as female includes how masculine or feminine a woman perceives herself to be and also how comfortable she is about her body image. The way the woman presents herself relates to how gender role-orientated she is in terms of wearing make-up, clothes etc. This definition has the benefit of including physiological, psychological and sociological aspects and the model relates to the western view of the world as well as to sexuality. It lacks discussion of how culture and society impinge on what is considered an acceptable sexual expression for women.

Female sexuality needs to be examined in the context of the historical, cultural, psychological, sociological and biological perspectives. Too many studies have been conducted which concentrate on only one aspect. This diminishes the reality of sexuality for the woman, who is affected in a unique way by all these perspectives. The adoption of a medical model for the study of sexuality can lead to pathologising events which, if seen in context, may be considered normal for the woman at that time. The removal of sexuality from childbirth and motherhood, creates a situation where the woman is seen as an asexual being, which can effect her transition to motherhood and put strain on the relationship with her sexual partner.

Historical and psychological perspectives

Female sexuality will be examined from the historical and psychological perspectives. A historical understanding of female sexuality explains where the theory originated that women were passive sexually, while men were active. The psychological perspective, particularly the psychoanalytical view, suggested that problems experienced by women could be explained by maladjustment in childhood resulting in 'penis envy'. Examination of the social construction of sexuality suggests that the examination of female sexuality from a scientific stance has removed it from the political arena.

Human sexuality has long been perceived as a very powerful force which required control. Predominately, this control was provided by rules and regulations laid down by both church and state (Haas and Haas, 1993). Women were seen as temptresses of men, allied with Satan and often in the guise of witches (Ussher, 1996). In Victorian times, it was believed that women could not enjoy sex, but viewed it as a dutiful role to be endured within marriage. Out of respect for their wives, therefore, Victorian males would only have coitus about once a month. Prostitution flourished and the double standards where 'nice' women did not enjoy sex and 'bad' women did, developed. Foucault (1976) states that this was linked to the emergence of capitalism. Sex once free and unfettered, was incompatible with the work ethic. Ussher (1996) states that, historically, female sexuality has been linked to reproduction. Women had either passive or voracious sexual appetites, but the aim remained procreation. She suggests that in the twentieth century, we have separated sex from reproduction so that sexual feelings in pregnant or lactating women are largely ignored within the medical press.

Jackson (1987) argues that when sexuality began to be viewed from a scientific perspective in the 1930s, it was removed from the sexual-political arena. Prior to this, women were fighting for sexual autonomy, which included control of their own sexuality free from male exploitation and coercion. With the emergence of the scientific view of sexuality, male sexual aggression and female passivity were deemed normal. Due to the high esteem in which science was held at the time, it was difficult to continue to challenge what feminists regarded as an issue of male dominance and power.

Freud proposed a developmental model of sexuality where an infant progressed through the oral, anal and genital phases until sexual maturity was reached (Haas and Haas, 1993). Each stage must be passed through or else development would be delayed. He put forward his theories of Oedipus and Electra to explain how males and females develop gender roles. While revolutionary in a time of repressed Victorian attitudes, the theories have been widely criticised, particularly by feminist writers. Oakley (1985) contends that male bias of unsupportable assumptions makes the theory open to criticisms. Why a girl should suffer from penis envy rather than a boy suffering from womb envy, or a girl should blame her mother but not her father because she has no penis has no logical basis. Siann (1996) asserts that psychoanalysts base their theories on clinical experience and case histories as opposed to empirical evidence. She also states that female cognitive psychologists have highlighted that most research findings were collected from male students by white middle-class researchers. This demonstrates how the ways in which evidence has been collected is being challenged in terms of the data being biased.

Llewelyn and Osborne (1990) discuss issues which affect women's sexual experiences. They suggest that for some women the context of their sexual experiences may be one of abuse and violence. Bewley and Gibbs (1994) contend that many women first experience domestic violence during pregnancy. Although Llewelyn and Osborne (1990) reject the concept that all men are sexual aggressors and all women are innocent victims, they contend that relationships between men and women can be improved. They describe how boys separate from their mothers by seeing the 'good mother' and the 'bad mother', thus setting up an arena for the struggle for power and control. This often leads to the setting up of sexual double standards where the woman is seen as either a mother or a whore.

An examination of the historical and psychological perspectives shows how the way female sexuality is viewed today is directly derived from theories from the past, many of which are now considered obsolete or open to challenge.

Biological perspective

The biological view of female sexuality took a scientific stance, monitoring the physiological aspects of woman's orgasms. Biological determinism concentrates on female sexuality for purposes of reproduction and the role sexuality has in keeping men and women together by providing for, and rearing, children.

Female sexuality has been examined under laboratory conditions by Masters and Johnson in the 1950s. From studying the biological data obtained, they developed a model of the female sexual response cycle. More recently, this has been modified by the American Psychiatric Association into DSM-IV (Bernhard, 1995). This consists of the appetitive, excitement, orgasm and resolution phases. The appetitive phase is mainly psychological leading to arousal; the excitement phase consists of physiological changes; the orgasm phase refers to the peak of sexual enjoyment and the resolution phase is when the body and mind return to a state of relaxation and a feeling of well-being. This model of sexual response may be criticised for not relating to women or girls who are unwilling performers during abusive or violent sexual assaults. Where is the 'feeling of well-being' during the resolution phase for these females? The generalisability of data obtained in the laboratory is questionable. The woman who volunteers to participate in coitus under these circumstances could not be said to be representative of all women. Penetrative sex is taken to be the norm, as is heterosexuality.

Studies relating to sexuality predominantly use the masculine norm, eg. coitus, to investigate female sexuality. This 'norm' includes the male right to coitus and the women as conforming. *The Hite Report* (1976) found that most women valued orgasm more than penetration. Ussher (1996) comments on a study which found that 80% of women report not having vaginal orgasm and requiring clitoral stimulation to climax. The myth of the vaginal orgasm stems from Freud, who believed that this was the 'adult orgasm' contrasting with the clitoral orgasm which was 'infantile' and should be abandoned (Wright, 1996). This has been described as 'psychological clitoridectomy'.

Similarities and differences between humans and non-human primates

Observational animal studies can be useful in illustrating the similarities and differences in human sexuality. Animals, such as monkeys, demonstrate that they are in a fertile period and ready to mate by physical changes which are overt biological signals to the male. Humans are capable of coitus at any time, although they are only fertile for about a week of each month. They are also likely to continue sexual activity throughout pregnancy, lactation and after the menopause (Pavelka, 1995). Sexual behaviour in women is not under hormonal control, so it may occur at random. However, human sexual activity does correspond to hormone activity. Studies show significant peaks in activity in mid-cycle, unless the woman is taking the contraceptive pill (Pavelka, 1995).

Wallen (1995) states that, although female sexual desire is clearly related to ovarian hormones, arousability to erotic stimuli is not. While arousability to erotic stimuli is similar for males and females, there appears to be a dearth of studies as to whether arousal-seeking behaviour between men and women is similar. Anecdotal evidence would say not, although this may be due to social perceptions of what normal sexual activity is for women, ie. of a more passive nature, where men are seen to actively seek sexual encounters (Wallen 1995). In one study Wellings *et al* (1994) found that 48.7% of men and 43.3% of women agreed strongly that orgasm is necessary to male sexual satisfaction, but a third of men disagreed. Thus, male orgasm is not universally perceived as necessary for male sexual satisfaction. This argues against all men being sexually aggressive. Male mammals normally attain ejaculatory behaviour, so this shows a basic difference between men and animals. It also warns against the reliability of extrapolating directly from animal studies to humans.

Although many female primates appear to be capable of achieving orgasm, it is clear coitus can be achieved without this. How important orgasm is to women is unclear. Some studies have shown that physical closeness and communication are the aspects of coitus that women value most (Wallen, 1995). Wellings et al (1994) found 37.4% of males and 28.6% of females thought that female orgasm was necessary for women's sexual satisfaction. This would suggest that men do not put their own sexual satisfaction first.

The following theory illustrates a direct relationship between the physiological changes which occur during coitus and lead to fertilisation.

Young (1993) reports on the 'upsuck' theory, which suggests that women control the amount of sperm retained following coitus by the timing of the female orgasm. If a woman does not have an orgasm or orgasms up to one minute before the man, she retains few sperm. If she orgasms within one minute of the man or up to forty five minutes after she retains a large number of sperm. This could effect the chances of her conceiving during coitus. Obviously this is dependent upon whether she was in the ovulatory phase of the fertility cycle, but this was not considered within the paper. It attempts to give a biological explanation for the female orgasm.

Non-human primates do not confine their sexual activities to heterosexual encounters and also have coitus during pregnancy. Sexual violence is another common factor shared between non-human primates and humans (Pavelka, 1995). Tuzin (1995) suggests that with humans there is a nearly universal need for privacy yet while having sex, we do not really know what people do.

The usefulness of studying animal behaviour in relation to sexuality is that it highlights an uninhibited sexuality unfettered by intelligent thought but nonetheless still sanctioned by the norms for the primate group.

None of the aspects considered so far are complete in themselves. If we take sexual development as a total of all those physical sensations which develop in infancy, eg. sucking at the breast, being bathed, stroked and cuddled, then sexuality for the adult female is more than coitus for reproduction (Llewelyn and Osborne, 1990). Van Wert (1991) suggests changing the emphasis in sexual relations from genital sex alone to embrace a wider context, which consists of sexual intimacies. These include: talking about life and sex, pampering each other with food, bathing together and enjoying sensual activities, such as touch, massage and suckling at the woman's breast.

Psychosocial aspects that may effect a woman's sexuality include her relationship with her sexual partner. If she is angry, upset or feels unsupported by her partner, she is unlikely to want to have sex (Curtis and Dunn, 1996). The continuum of childbearing as well as preconceptional life experiences for both partners integrate to impact on the sexuality of both women and their partners. Men and women are affected by the transitions to parenthood. In the postpartum period the woman is making the transition to motherhood and also coping with changes in the relationship with her partner.

Cultural perspective

When studying female sexuality, it is necessary to remember that it is always expressed in a cultural context. Although the physiological mechanisms may be the same for all women, the cultural context may vary. The cultural norm in western society would be female sexual expression within a heterosexual relationship, linked with procreation. In fact, this stereotypic approach denies the expression of sexuality along a continuum ranging from celibacy, women alone, lesbians, bisexuality, to heterosexual behaviour (Bernhard, 1995). The expression of sexuality consists of a variety of behaviour including masturbation, oral sex, coitus, voyeurism, exhibitionism, sadomasochism, fetishism, group sex etc.

In many cultural groups, female virginity is seen as important not only for moral and religious reasons, but also for the economic benefits such a woman will bring to her family in terms of a dowry. It ensures (in theory) that family wealth passing down the male line, goes to the biological offspring of the father. Brody (1988) states that in all cultural groups women have controlled their own fertility by using a variety of methods to avoid conception or terminate unwanted pregnancy. As young women will not be available to young men, some cultural groups encourage adolescent boys to form sexual relationships with older men until marriage. Among the Nyakyusa society in Africa, premarital sexual relationships among males and females are accepted (Schlegel 1995). In Bastar, central India, the Muria tribe adolescents have sexual relationships within their local area. Changing partners is encouraged, to prevent too intense relationships within pairs that are not sanctioned to marry. This data indicates that sexuality is socially constructed not biologically innate.

In developing countries, women are still subject to patriarchy and male control of their sexual and reproductive functions. These are largely linked with lack of education and employment opportunities among women. In industrial societies where these have improved for women, it is accepted that women have wider roles within society than the sexual and reproductive aspects. They are accepted as useful members of society, even when they choose to remain childless or are childless due to infertility (Brody, 1988).

Is childbirth sexual?

The aim of this chapter is to highlight the themes of the type of research which has been conducted into childbirth and sexuality. The similarities of the physiological responses that occur in coitus, labour and breast-feeding will be examined. The psychological and physiological effects of sexual symbolism and imagery on labour in different cultural groups will be discussed, and finally the debate between breast-feeding and sexual response will be examined.

A review of the literature examining sexuality and childbirth highlights certain themes. Sexuality in pregnancy examines whether coitus may stimulate uterine contractions (Moore et al, 1994, Brustman et al, 1989), what rates of sexual interest and coitus in pregnancy may be considered average (El-Tomi et al, 1993, Frohlich et al, 1990), the risk of premature rupture of the membranes (PROM) during coitus (Ekwo et al, 1993), what infections may occur as a result of coitus in pregnancy (Kurki and Ylikorkala, 1993; Read and Klebanoff, 1993) and what sexual problems may occur (Reamy and White, 1985).

Sex and sexual difficulties after childbirth exist in relation to the timing of resumption of coitus, problems with resumption of coitus (Sarrel and Sellgren, 1992), problems with male sexuality following childbirth (O' Driscoll, 1994) and resumption of coitus, particularly looking at the type of suture materials used in the event of perineal tears or episiotomy (Grant, 1989; Mahomed et al, 1989) or the social aspects of episiotomy (Sleep, 1990; Kitzinger, 1990, Barrett and Victor, 1996). The majority of research overwhelmingly adheres to a male model of sexuality, ignoring what women have to say about their own understanding of sexuality and the many dimensions which relate to it (Kitzinger, 1995). These themes also reflect aspects of sexuality where couples are likely to receive conflicting advice from healthcare professionals (Sarrel and Sellgren, 1992). Adherence to a medical model of childbirth makes it understandable that the way that sexuality has been studied also uses a medical model. It is rarely acknowledged that the way maternity care is given may cause the problems with sexuality from which some women suffer.

Walton (1994), O'Driscoll (1994) and Curtis and Dunn (1996) embrace a biopsychosocial model of childbirth and examine sexuality and childbirth from a multidimensional perspective. This includes a comprehensive understanding of the physiological changes in childbirth which effect sexuality, especially the hormonal factors. The psychological, social and cultural aspects of each woman will affect her individual sexual experience during childbirth. This appears to offer a meaningful examination of sexuality.

Walton (1997) argues that sexuality is a state of being and cannot be separated from childbirth. 'It is concerned with sexual orientation, desires, expressiveness, innate feelings, sexual instincts and identity at every stage of the lifespan. This being so, the childbearing year is no exception and, in fact, sexuality impinges on the process for the women, their partners and their carers to an extent which is not always recognised.'

Different cultural practices, which concern abstaining from coitus during pregnancy, appear to stem from the knowledge that babies do not always survive the pregnancy, and there is a supposition that this may be connected with coitus. The taboos against coitus continue in developed countries, despite advances in scientific knowledge which contradict the need for abstinence. This may be demonstrated in the inaccurate advice given to pregnant women by some healthcare professionals in the western world (Sarrel and Sellgren, 1992).

Conception in most instances is the result of a sexual act. There are similar physiological responses found in coitus, labour and breast-feeding. The hormone, oxytocin, which is secreted from the posterior lobe of the pituitary gland and is released during orgasm, labour and breast-feeding, acts on the smooth muscle of the uterus and makes it contract rhythmically (McNabb, 1997). The plasma level of the neurohormone, endorphin, is raised during orgasm, labour and breast-feeding, and induces a feeling of well-being and relieves pain. Midwives know that nipple stimulation or masturbation can be used by the woman and her partner to accelerate labour by stimulating the release of oxytocin (Robinson, 1991). Some women experience sexual response during labour (Gaskin, 1988). One midwife reports of a woman pleading to be masturbated (by the student midwife) during the second stage of labour (Southern, 1994).

Many cultural groups use sexual symbolism and imagery to provide psychological support to women during labour (Bates and Turner, 1985). Young male mountain dwellers from a village in Burma, pose naked in obscene postures in front of a labouring woman to embarrass and frighten away evil spirits. The father of the unborn baby strips naked and exposes his genitalia to induce labour in the Mbuti pygmy culture of Central Africa and the Arunta of Central

Australia. Drinking water in which her husband's loincloth had been washed is used to treat prolonged and difficult labour experienced by women in rural Delhi. Women in Jamaica sniff a sweaty shirt worn by a man to speed up labour. The sexual imagery may provoke a sexual response in the woman, leading to physiological changes which may effect labour as the hormones released in coitus and labour are the same (Bates and Turner, 1985).

In western societies, the emphasis on the breast as a sexual object has affected some women to the extent that they choose not to breast-feed their babies. Some women feel uncomfortable going against society's norms by breast-feeding. Others have problems with their partners' sexual jealousy, which is exacerbated by their breast-feeding. The belief by some people that breast-feeding may induce sexual feelings or orgasm is a reason why some women choose not to breast feed (Rodriguez-Garcia and Frazier, 1995).

Newton (1975) states that similarities which occur in both coitus and breast-feeding are the contraction of the uterus, nipple erection, breast stimulation and a change in blood flow to the skin. She argues that society tries to deny the sexual aspect of breast-feeding. Part of her argument is based on findings of studies which purported to show that women who breast-fed were more at ease with their sexuality and resumed coitus sooner after the birth than bottle-feeders. Kayner and Zagar (1983) contest this view in a study of 121 lactating women. This found that 62.6% of the women reported less or no sexual desire while breast-feeding than before birth, 26.1% had the same level of desire and 11.3% had more sexual desire.

Walton (1994) states that the suggestion that women experience orgasm while breast-feeding is a sinister myth. She maintains that what women experience emotionally while breast-feeding is very different from the emotions of coitus. Physiologically, oxytocin is released by the mother's pituitary gland during breast-feeding, on seeing, thinking, or hearing her child. Together with prolactin, these hormones contribute to feelings of maternal well-being in nursing mothers and sensual pleasures. Oxytocin 'the hormone of love' is also released during coitus (Newton, 1978). The link between the sexual act and breast-feeding may cause pleasure to one women and shame and disgust to another. Clearly, the physiological cannot be separated from the psychological and cultural perception of what is acceptable. The debate centres on whether society is repressing women by denying the sexual nature of breast-feeding or whether suggesting a sexual element is demeaning a nurturing act and linking it with child abuse. Reflecting on the individual experience of sexuality and the lack of research into this question, there is no clear conclusion to this argument at this time. Is there confusion about the sensual experience of breast-feeding with sexual experience or is the sensual experience part of the sexual continuum? Alternatively, is it simply that the definitions of sexuality by individuals and society result in narrow parameters which fail to accept and embrace its complex nature.

Most cultural groups have a period of sexual abstinence of one to two months in the postpartum period (Sarrel and Sellgren, 1992). Traditional African-Caribbean women may wait until the lochia has stopped, Akan (Ghanaian) women may wait three months and Somali women may wait 40 days to resume coitus (Schott and Henley, 1996). Some religious groups also have restrictions over the resumption of sexual intercourse. Jewish and Hindu women may wait until the lochia has stopped and Muslim women may also wait 40 days. Whether for cultural or religious reasons, sexual abstinence usually relates to a belief that a woman who is menstruating or has lochia present is unclean. Christian women do not have special restrictions (Schott and Henley, 1996).

The many reasons why one could argue that childbirth is sexual include: that sexuality is an integral part of the human state, procreation is usually the result of coitus, and childbirth itself is an event which affects the sexual organs. Women continue to have coitus throughout pregnancy and sexual stimulation is known to have a favourable effect on labour. The similarity of physiological responses during coitus, labour and breast-feeding is also significant. The debate concerning the issue of breast-feeding and sexual response continues.

Women who require special consideration during childbirth

This section focuses on two groups of women: adult survivors of sexual abuse and lesbians. Women from these groups are absent from models of female sexuality. Their special needs are ignored when receiving maternity care, unless they choose to disclose a history of past sexual abuse or lesbianism. Many healthcare professionals are unaware of caring for women from these groups although they make up a sizeable percentage of the population.

Survivors of sexual abuse or rape

It is important to consider how sexual abuse and violence may effect the childbearing woman. Because the experience of sexual abuse may never be disclosed, it is not possible to be precise about its prevalence. Figures previously cited include 1:4 women (Lecky-Thompson, 1995) or 20% of women (Mullen, 1991; in Reece, 1996). It is possible that any woman cared for by a midwife has been subjected to some form of sexual abuse or violence (Parratt, 1994). Midwives do not routinely ask pregnant women if they have a past history of sexual abuse or violence, although it could affect their experience of childbirth. Most of the literature in relation to abuse and childbirth is anecdotal and unreferenced.

Some of the anecdotal evidence (Lecky-Thompson, 1995; Burian, 1995) indicates that women may remember past sexual abuse during pregnancy or childbirth. Parratt (1994) discusses the psychological theory that views pregnancy as a developmental life event that leads to re-examination of issues surrounding previous abuse. Another perspective is that childbirth itself has many psychological aspects which may trigger memories of past abuse. Studies have not been done to ascertain if midwives find that women choose to disclose this information or whether it is more likely to occur at a particular time in childbirth.

Some papers have compiled characteristics which might lead a midwife to suspect that a woman has been abused. These include not wanting a male carer, over-dependence or no connection with the labour partner, difficulty discussing feelings and difficulties with breast-feeding (Shelby Wescott, 1991). These seem somewhat vague and imprecise. Parratt (1994) in a study of six survivors of childhood sexual abuse found that issues relating to privacy, control and touch were important for these women's childbirth experiences. Kitzinger (1992) states that women who have been sexually abused in childhood often compare the experience of childbirth in the terminology of rape. Other concerns relate to the potential abuse of the new baby by the mother or others.

She also discusses the prospect that staff may treat a woman in a paternalistic fashion or infantilise her while penetrative and painful medical procedures are performed. A medicalised approach to childbirth subjects women to routine assaults on the body and the mind. They may be translated as necessary interventions aimed at safeguarding the health and well-being of mother and child. For example, numerous vaginal examinations, the application of a fetal scalp electrode, amniotomy in labour and, finally, the act of giving birth itself can be abusive and traumatic to victims of abuse. Additionally, the language linked to the explanations given prior to procedures could be construed as an assault if it echoes past abuse experiences for women.

Women survivors of sexual abuse have been noted for 'dissociation' while in labour (Burian, 1995). This may assist the woman to cope with pain, by becoming detached from her body. Burian states that we must help ground the woman and make her aware of her surroundings. This would appear to be an unresearched approach. It is unclear why a potentially useful coping strategy should be challenged during labour.

Studies have shown that an increased number of women receiving treatment for psychiatric disorders have had past experience of sexual abuse (Walker and James, 1992). Reece (1996) maintains that women receiving psychiatric care for self-harm behaviour sometimes have a history of previous sexual abuse. She states that women who have been sexually abused have been victims of patriarchy in the home and also suffer from a patriarchal system offering psychiatric care. The majority of women working as prostitutes were sexually abused as children (Benson and Matthews, 1995). This suggests that women survivors of sexual abuse may benefit from professional help which allows them to work through past events and come to terms with it as best they can.

For those women who choose to disclose previous sexual abuse, it is hoped that midwives could use a sensitive approach to their care which 'counteracts rather than re-enacts the violation of women's bodies' (Kitzinger, 1992). As most women apparently choose not to disclose, care of all women should bear in mind a potential past history of abuse. Women should be treated with respect and permission sought prior to touching her or her baby. Ensuring privacy and assisting women to remain in control during childbirth should result from an individualised approach to care (Parratt, 1994). Midwives need to devise better methods of supporting these women by learning more about how individual women feel.

Lesbians

Although lesbians make up between 2–12% of the female population (Zeidenstein, 1990), their existence and special needs are infrequently acknowledged within the childbirth arena. They have unique needs arising from the chosen method of conception, inappropriate health advise based on an assumption of heterosexuality, non-inclusion of the supportive partner in care and a lack of understanding of the types of parenting problems which they may encounter. Some midwives and doctors may never be aware that some of their clients are lesbians.

How lesbians become pregnant has significant implications for health. Coitus with a man who has agreed to help father a child or who may be unsuspecting, may put the woman at risk of sexually transmitted diseases or human immunodeficiency virus (HIV) or acquired immunodeficiency syndrome (AIDS) (Zeidenstein, 1990). A woman may conceive following self-administered insemination of sperm which may or may not have been screened for disease. Lesbians may have received sperm donations from male homosexual friends, sometimes with the intention of raising the child together. In order to prevent identification of the sperm donor and possible later claims of paternity rights, the woman may choose to use multiple donors (Wismont and Reame, 1989). All of these methods carry health risks. Wismont and Reame suggest that donor insemination assists with the acceptance of the pregnancy for the lesbian couple, possibly due to the careful planning required. Active involvement in the process by the partner is to be encouraged.

Once pregnant, a lesbian may choose not to disclose her sexual orientation to healthcare professionals. This may result in inappropriate information-gathering by the midwife, for example queries about previous contraception use (Wilton, 1996). Inappropriate assumptions about the client's heterosexuality may lead the midwife to exclude the lesbian's female partner from participating in her care, casting her in the role of a friend and the pregnant woman into the role of a single parent when this may not be the case. This has implications for labour when the intimate support of her lover may be important to the pregnant woman and yet may take on a covert role when the midwife is present. This may influence the woman's choice of place of birth, as she may feel more able to be in control in her own home (Tash and Kenney, 1993). Midwives, unaware of the true nature of the relationship between the couple, may deprive the non-biological parent of opportunities to properly bond with the baby from the start.

Parenting issues for the lesbian may include worries about bonding with a male infant (Zeidenstein, 1990) and how the lesbian couple choose to parent their baby. The biological parent will have legal rights over the baby and may want to consider transferring those to her partner to show commitment to the relationship. This will depend very much on each individual couple's relationship. Lesbian couples may have fears that someone may try to take the baby away from them through the courts, as has happened on some occasions (Wismont and Reame, 1989) and lesbians may feel more supported by their friends than by their families. There are differing views among lesbians about the appropriateness of parenthood for lesbians, which may also cause concern to the new parents. What role will the non-biological parent take in child-rearing? Will the child have two mothers? For some lesbian couples both partners will breast-feed the baby. This is an important health consideration for lesbians, as the risk of breast cancer is increased in women who do not breast-feed (Zeidenstein, 1990). These are all issues which lesbian couples will need to consider and from which they could benefit by having open discussion with sensitive and informed healthcare professionals.

Lack of awareness by healthcare professionals that women in their care may be lesbians prevents these women from receiving optimum care. Wilton (1996) suggests that education of midwives should include how to set the scene whereby lesbians may feel comfortable in disclosing their sexual orientation and not feel fearful that their care may be adversely affected by disclosure. This may include not assuming that all women are heterosexual and phrasing questions during history-taking in a way that acknowledges this. Individual women have the right not to disclose, but setting up an open environment where women feel safe to do so may improve the care to this group. Midwives need to come to terms with their own sexuality and have their views of others challenged rigorously before they can meaningfully support clients of a different sexual orientation.

Conclusion

Female sexuality is diverse. For too long we have shied away from the sexual aspects of childbirth. This has resulted in poor care for pregnant women. Part of this may have been the direct result of inadequate understanding of female sexuality. A wider approach to female sexuality should include discussion of its social construction and the effect of outdated attitudes which originated in Victorian times. Over-reliance on the objectivity of a masculine-dominated scientific approach has produced a narrow understanding of physiological responses of the sexual act, as if one can set this apart from the individual woman's feelings, beliefs and past experiences. Examples from different cultural groups make it clear that an ethnocentric or heterosexual framework for sexual expression, is only an example of one type of sexual life. The deficit in understanding here completes a continuum in which female sexuality has been splintered into meanings which suit masculine perceptions of women and masculine approaches to childbearing.

References

Barrett G, Victor C (1996) Incidence of postnatal dyspareunia. *Br J Sex Med* September/October: 6–8

Bates B, Turner AN (1985) Imagery and symbolism in the birth practices of traditional cultures. *Birth* **12**(1): 29–35

Benson C, Matthews R (1995) Street prostitution: Ten facts in search of a policy. *Int J Sociol Law* **23**(4):394–415

Bernhard LA (1995) Sexuality in women's lives. In: Fogel CI, Woods NF, eds. *Women's Healthcare*. Sage Publications, London: 475–95

Bewley C, Gibbs A (1994) Coping with domestic violence in pregnancy. *Nurs Stand* **8**(50):25–8

Brody EB (1988) Culture, reproductive technology and women's rights: an intergovernmental perspective. *J Psychosom Obstet Gynaecol* **9**: 199–205

Brustman LE, Raptoulis M, Langer O *et al* (1989) Changes in the pattern of uterine contractility in relationship to coitus during pregnancies at low and high risk for preterm labour. *Obstet Gynaecol* **73**(2): 166–8

Burian J (1995) Helping survivors of sexual abuse through labour. *Am J Mat/Child Nurs* **20**(5): 252–6

Curtis P, Dunn K (1996) Sex and sexuality. *Mod Midwife* **May**: 26–9

Ekwo EE, Gosselink CA, Woolson R *et al* (1993) Coitus late in pregnancy: risk of preterm rupture of amniotic sac membranes. *Am J Obstet Gynecol* **168**(1): 22–31

El-Tomi NF, Bustan M AL, Abokhadour N (1992–3) Maternal sexuality during pregnancy and after childbirth in Kuwait. *Int Q Comm Health Educ* **13**(2):163–73

Foucault M (1976) *The History of Sexuality: An Introduction*, Vol 1. Penguin Books, London

Frohlich EP, Herz C, van der Merwe FJ (1990) Sexuality during pregnancy and early puerperium and its perception by the pregnant and puerperal woman. *J Psychosom Obstet Gynaecol* **11**: 73–80

Gaskin IM (1988) Ask the midwife. *Birth Gaz* **4**(2): 27

Grant A (1989) The choice of suture materials and techniques for repair of perineal trauma: an overview of the evidence from controlled trials. *Br J Obstet Gynaecol* **96**(11): 1281–9

Haas K, Haas A (1993) *Understanding Sexuality*, 3rd edn. Mosby, St. Louis

Hite S (1976) *The Hite Report*. Macmillan, New York

Jackson M (1987) 'Facts of life' or the eroticization of women's oppression? Sexology and the social construction of heterosexuality. In: Caplan P, ed. *The Cultural Construction of Sexuality*. Routledge, London

Kayner CE, Zagar JA (1983) Breast-feeding and sexual response. *J Fam Pract* **17**(1): 69–73

Kitzinger J (1992) Counteracting, not re-enacting, the violation of women's bodies: the challenge for perinatal caregivers. *Birth* **19**(4): 219–20

Kitzinger S (1990) Episiotomy, body image and sex. In: Kitzinger S, Simkin P, eds. *Episiotomy and the Second Stage of Labour*. Pennypress, Seattle:102–8

Kitzinger S (1995) MIDIRS abstract in MIDIRS. *Midwif Digest* **Dec**: 451

Kurki T, Ylikorkala O (1993) Coitus during pregnancy is not related to bacterial vaginosis or preterm birth. *Am J Obstet Gynecol* **169**(5): 1130–4

Lecky-Thompson M (1995) Surviving childhood sexual abuse: what is the midwife's role? *Communique* **6**(3): 15–16

Llewelyn S, Osborne K (1990) *Women's Lives*. Routledge, London

Mahomed K, Grant A, Ashurst H *et al* (1989) A randomized comparison of suture materials and suturing techniques for repair of perineal trauma. *Br J Obstet Gynaecol* **96**(11):1272–80

McNabb M (1997) Hormonal interactions in labour. In: Sweet BR, ed. *Mayes Midwifery*, 12th edn. Bailliere Tindall, London: 343–54

Moore TR, Iams JD, Creasy RK *et al* (1994) Diurnal and gestational patterns of uterine activity in normal human pregnancy. *Obstet Gynecol* **83**(4): 517–23

Mullen PE (1994) Consequences of childhood sexual abuse. *Br Med J* **303**: 144–5

Newton M (1975) Trebly sensuous woman. *Psychology Today* **1**: 33–5

Newton N (1978) The role of oxytocin reflexes in three interpersonal reproductive acts: Coitus, birth and breastfeeding. In: Carenza L, Panceri P, Zichella L eds. *Clinical Psychoneuroendocrinology in Reproduction*. Proceedings of the Serona Symposia, Vol 22. Academic Press, New York: 411–18

Oakley A (1985) *Sex, Gender and Society*. Gower Publishing, Aldershot

O'Driscoll M (1994) Midwives, childbirth and sexuality. *Br J Midwif* **2**(1): 39 41

Parratt J (1994) The experience of childbirth for survivors of incest. *Midwifery* **10**: 26–39

Pavelka MSM (1995) Sexual nature: what can we learn from a cross-species perspective? In: Abramson PR, Pinkerton ST, eds. *Sexual Nature, Sexual Culture*. University of Chicago Press, Chicago: 17–36

Pinkola EC (1994) *Women Who Run with the Wolves: Contacting the Power of the Wild Women*. Rider and Co, London

Read JS, Klebanoff MA (1993) Sexual intercourse during pregnancy and preterm delivery: effects of vaginal micro-organisms. *Am J Obstet Gynecol* **168**(2): 514–19

Reamy KJ, White SE (1985) Dyspareunia in pregnancy. *J Psychosom Obstet Gynaecol* **4**: 263–70

Reece J (1996) Patriarchal power and the female sexual abuse survivor. The medicalisation of the body. Unpublished article

Robinson J (1991) Sexuality and birth. *Homebirth Aus Newsletter* **29**:11–16

Rodriguez-Garcia R, Frazier L (1995) Cultural paradoxes relating to sexuality and breastfeeding. *J Hum Lact* **11**(2): 111–14

Sarrel PM, Sellgren UM (1992) Sexuality in pregnancy and the puerperium. In: Reece EA, Hobbins JC, Mahoney MJ *et al*, eds. *Medicine of the Fetus and Mother*. JP Lippincott, Philadelphia: 1285–92

Schlegel A (1995) The cultural management of adolescent sexuality. In: Abramson PR, Pinkerton SD, eds. *Sexual Nature, Sexual Culture*. University of Chicago Press, Chicago: 177–94

Schott J, Henley A (1996) *Culture, Religion and Childbearing in a Multiracial Society*. Butterworth Heinmann, Oxford

Shelby Wescott C (1991) Sexual abuse and childbirth education. *IJCE* **November**: 32–3

Siann G (1996) Gender and gender identity. In: Niven CA, Walker A, eds. *Reproductive Potential and Fertility Control*. Butterworth-Heinemann, Oxford: 1–15

Sleep J (1990) Episiotomy. In: Faulkner A, Murphy-Black T, eds. *Midwifery*. Scutari Press, Harrow: 7–18

Southern M (1994) Labour and sexuality. *Midwifery Matters*. **61**: 5–7

Tash DT, Kenney JW (1993) The lesbian childbearing couple: a case report. *Birth* **20**(1): 36–40

Tuzin D (1995) Discourse, intercourse, and the excluded middle: anthropology and the problem of sexual experience. In: *Sexual Nature, Sexual Culture*. University of Chicago Press. Chicago: 257–75

Ussher JM (1993) *The Psychology of the Female Body*. Routledge, London

Ussher JM (1996) Female sexuality and reproduction. In: Niven CA, Walker A, eds. *Reproductive Potential and Fertility Control*. Butterworth-Heinemann, Oxford

Van Wert WF (1991) Sex after children. *Mothering*. **60**: 115–17

Walker S, James H (1992) Childhood physical and sexual abuse in women. *Psychiatry Pract* **Spring**: 15–18

Wallen K (1995) Evolution of female sexual desire. In: Abramson PR, Pinkerton SD, eds. *Sexual Nature, Sexual Culture*. University of Chicago Press. Chicago: 57–79.

Walton I (1994) *Sexuality and Motherhood*. Books for Midwives Press, Altrincham

Walton I (1997) Sexuality and childbearing. In: Sweet BR, ed. *Mayes Midwifery,* 12th edn. Bailliere Tindall, London: 741–7

Wellings K, Field J, Johnson AM, Wadsworth J (1994) *Sexual Behaviour in Britain*. Penguin Books, Harmondsworth

Wilton T (1996) Caring for the lesbian client: homophobia and midwifery. *Br J Midwif* **4**(3): 126–31

Wismont JM, Reame NE (1989) The lesbian childbearing experience: assessing developmental tasks. *IMAGE: J Nurs Schol* **21**(3): 137–41

Wright J (1996) Female genital mutilation: an overview. *J Adv Nurs* **24**: 251–9

Young S (1993) The subtle side of sex. *New Sci* **August 14**: 24–7

Zeidenstein L (1990) Gynecological and childbearing needs of lesbians. *J Nurse-Midwif* **35**(1):10–18

Part 2
Meeting the needs of specific client groups

5
Healthcare for lesbian, gay, and bisexual individuals

Matthew V Morrissey

This chapter will examine issues in relation to healthcare for lesbian, gay or bisexual clients focusing on areas, such as homosexuality and society, public opinion and public policy. A brief history of homosexuality and healthcare, law, religion and homosexuality, and attitudes of health professionals to clients who are lesbian, gay or bisexual is also included. It will be shown that health professionals are in a key position to promote respect and 'depathologise' same-sex relationships. It is hoped that such a discussion will stimulate dialogue and improve health professionals' confidence, knowledge and sensitivity.

History, homosexuality and society

'Are you gay or straight?'

The above quote, although seemingly harmless, identifies some need in western society to 'pigeon hole' or alienate people on grounds of their sexual orientation. Historically, the characteristic horror of homosexuality in western culture dates back to the fourteenth century. Although most societies have sexual taboos, and many of them apply to certain forms of same-sex behaviour (or even to all same-sex erotic activity), few if any major cultures have made homosexuality — either as a general classification act according to gender, or as an 'orientation' — the primary and singular moral taboo it has long been in western society: 'the sin that cannot be named', 'the unmentionable vice,' 'the love that dare not speak its name' (Boswell, 1996). Those who never had occasion to question this extraordinary prejudice, especially if they personally entertain reservations about homosexual acts, may have difficulty apprehending how remarkable this degree of revulsion actually is. Murder, matricide, child molesting, incest, cannibalism, genocide, even deicide are topics for general discussion: why, therefore, are a few disapproved sexual acts that injure no one so much more horrible than these? Because they are worse? In fact, no moral system of general application in the west would actually categorise homosexual relations between consenting adults as worse than child molesting (which is now commonly discussed). It is the affective taboo aspect of the subject which rendered it unmentionable until recently. There are many positive stories about same-sex relationships from a rich and positive past casting dismay on modern superficial discourse. For example Iolaus who shared the Labours of Hercules and fought by his side, was beloved by him. Aristotle says that even down to his day (fourth century BC) the tomb of Iolaus was a place where same-sex lovers plighted mutual faith. Centuries before, Plato had put the same idea in the mouth of Aristophanes, who claimed that males who preferred other males and 'delight to lie with them to be clasped in men's embraces . . . are the finest boys and young men, for they have the most manly nature . . . Their behaviour is due to daring manliness and virility, since they are quick to welcome their like' (Boswell, 1996). The Greeks idealised love between an older male mentor and a younger male student. In a late classical novel involving a lengthy dispute over whether it is better for men to love other men or women, the proponent of the former having argued that same-sex loves are the 'most stable' of erotic passions, expresses the hope that he will be buried with his lover after they have passed their lives together (Lucian, cited in Macleod, 1967). Doubtless the most surprising and counterintuitive aspect of Greek same-sex eroticism was not its frequency or duration, but its long and hallowed relationship to democracy and military valour, which modern military officials find improbable or even unbelievable (Boswell, 1996).

Roman same-sex relationships have been less well studied. On the one hand there is the idealised and formal lover/beloved relationships imputed to the Greeks and on the other the riotous and promiscuous sexuality which forms such a lurid mythology about the Roman Empire.

However, contrary to many accounts by imperial literature, there were also many same-sex couples of both sexes in the Roman world who lived together permanently, forming unions neither more nor less exclusive than those of the heterosexual couples around them. The irony in present times is that many people remain ignorant of the nature of relationships of lesbian, gay and bisexual people. Indeed many people may find it threatening that two women or two men can form loving as well as sexual relationships. More importantly, the heterosexual/homosexual distinction as a construction inhibits appreciation of the diversity of human experience by encouraging use of static labels to classify individuals' continually evolving sexual histories (Epting *et al*, 1994). Sexual categories which seem so obvious to us now and divide humanity into 'heterosexuals' and 'homosexuals', appear to have been unknown in ancient times. However, such a dichotomy is inaccurate given that a proportion of society is bisexual. In fact the term 'homosexual' was only introduced in the nineteenth century.

Throughout history, with few exceptions, lesbians have either been ignored or tolerated, while male homosexuals have received most of the condemnation (Carlson, 1990). According to Bullough (1979), 'This double standard may have existed so long because the males who have dominated the writing of history and the making of laws have assumed that women were nothing without men, and that no sex could take place without a penis involved'. Sadly, there is much ignorance surrounding the history and sexuality of women who define themselves as lesbian. Lesbian women do not wish to be seen as having forsworn their womanhood, as loving women because they are bent on revenge against men, or as having no desire for a man's love and the love of children (Magee and Miller, 1994).

Historically, homosexuality has always existed in spite of varying degrees of persecution, oppression, legislation and other forms of social control (Davies and Neal, 1996). In general, it has been found that four to six percent of the population, both women and men, are exclusively homosexual (Meyer, 1985).

In a cross-cultural study by Sell *et al* (1990) concerning same-sex sexual behaviour of men, 11.6% of French and American men, and 7.8% of British men reported same-sex sexual behaviour from the age of fifteen. Furthermore, 10.8% of French men, 4.7% of British men and 6.3% of American men reported same-sex sexual behaviour within the previous five years. To have a homosexual encounter is one thing but to be exclusively homosexual is entirely different (Davies and Neal, 1996). What is clear is that many individuals are bisexual. However, homosexuality occurs in all cultures (Weinrich and Williams, 1991).

Same-sex orientation is a fundamental form of human sexuality acted out in different cultural settings (Carlson, 1990). Even though same-sex orientation may not be a creation of social structure, such structure has a powerful influence on relationships in everyday life, including the expression of sexuality, friendship, affection and love. Negative attitudes and the prejudice of society towards homosexuality is sometimes expressed when a partner dies, as the following examples illustrate.

Barry and David had a long-standing homosexual relationship, but when David became terminally ill and was admitted to the intensive care unit of his local hospital, his family were at his bedside and refused to let Barry visit. So David and Barry never got a chance to say goodbye to one another and, when it came to the funeral, David's family made it quite clear that Barry was not welcome there either. If a heterosexual partner dies, everyone is sympathetic, but when a homosexual partner dies, the one remaining can face hostility, not empathy (Wertheimer, 1987).

Mary's problems began after her partner died. She and Betty had lived together for over twenty years and they were running a nursing home for elderly people when Betty died. The home was in a small village; no one else in the local community knew about their lesbian relationship and so it was assumed Mary had simply lost her business partner. Faced with the loss of her lover, and the subsequent loss of home and livelihood, Mary had no one to turn to. Even worse, on the day of the funeral, she still had to go on caring for the elderly residents of the home unable publicly to acknowledge the nature and magnitude of her loss (Wertheimer, 1987).

Public policy and opinion remain important areas in shaping and controlling the expression of same-sex relationships, to such an extent that the expression of mild affectionate gestures in public can result in violent attacks for gay men (Rivers, 1996).

Public opinion and public policy

Recently, it has been suggested that there is increasing tolerance of gay and lesbian people in western countries who 'openly wear the badge of homosexuality' (Campion, 1995). However, few studies if any identify whether there is any real substance to this tolerance given that many gay men have been the victims of gross human rights violations (Sieghart, 1989; Cohen, 1997), homophobia (Tierney, 1995; Morrissey, 1996), aggression and violence (Morrow, 1993) and bullying in UK schools (Rivers, 1996). Doctors have lost their jobs because of their sexual orientation (Rose, 1994) and there continues to be inequality in the age of consent in the UK. In the UK and the USA, gay men and lesbian women are seeking equality in their public and private lives. In the USA, it has been demonstrated that the public has become less willing to endorse proposals to restrict homosexuals' expression of their ideas through public speeches, teaching in colleges, and placement in public libraries of books written by gay authors. In contradiction to this, it was found that moral judgments about homosexuality have become more negative (Dejowski, 1992).

In America, hatred and misunderstanding in the public discussion of homosexuality seems to have increased some gay and lesbian youths' distress and interfered with their psychosexual functioning (Kleis and Lock, 1995). In the UK, there is conflict in public policy in relation to same-sex relationships, and in some local authorities there are initiatives to create tolerance of homosexuality. However, central government legislation, such as *Section 28* of the 1988 *Local Government Act*, makes it illegal for local authorities to 'promote the teaching in any maintained school of the acceptability of homosexuality as a pretend family relationship' (Campion, 1995).

Coming to terms with sexuality and identity may be a real struggle for young people who often lack role models, and social support (Rotheram *et al*, 1995). Much of the literature outlines this process as 'coming out' when individuals are coming to terms with being gay, lesbian or bisexual (Magee and Miller, 1994). However, there is very little evidence that such a process offers a simple set formula in integrating sexual orientation with self-identity. There are different issues for young people to come to terms with as they grow and develop. For many young and old, the concept of coming out is fundamental to personal identity and being part of a larger group. The process of coming out becomes a central developmental task and a challenge in the search of personal identity (Rotheram *et al*, 1995). However, acceptance or non-acceptance by others will not necessarily bring about positive acceptance of self. Rather more time should be spent on offering affirmative support and education for young people on relationships and sexuality. In education, role play may be a useful tool for young men and women in exploring issues to do with the process of coming out (Walters and Phillips, 1994).

It has also been suggested that much variation in 'being out' can be explained by factors, such as income, occupation, where one lives and the nature of one's friends, rather than as a stage of the coming out process (Joseph, 1993). It has also been argued that there are common situations in which it is not morally appropriate to come out or be out at all (Barbone and Rice, 1994). It is important to appreciate that many individuals may only come to terms with aspects of their sexuality and identity when they are in a close, loving relationship. Lack of sensitivity can bring about dire consequences. Suicide is sometimes the sad result for some teenagers unable to cope with their confusion, and the stigma surrounding their sexual orientation (Millard, 1995; Nelson, 1997). This may also be intensified by victimisation and bullying at school (Rivers 1996).

If the reality is that homosexuality is taboo at school and at home, and young people may be rejected by parents if they 'come out' (Morrow, 1993), where can the teenager get help? In recent years the AIDS education charity, AVERT, has attempted to address these issues by producing resources on sexual issues for young people and teachers (Clift *et al*, 1996; 1997), a leaflet on 'Young gay men talking' (Frankham and Kanabus, 1996) and a resource to support teachers talking about homosexuality in the secondary school (Forrest *et al*, 1997).

Many telephone help lines now operate including gay and lesbian switchboards which offer advice, support and information about groups in local areas in the UK. Counselling is also available from a number of agencies that often advertise locally and in the gay press. Although some believe that homosexuality is now more acceptable (Gallop

Report, 1982; Carlson, 1990; Campion, 1995), many professionals and a large section of the public continue to have negative and judgmental attitudes towards such relationships (Morrissey, 1996). Recently a curriculum has been put forward in relation to teaching about lesbian, gay and bisexual issues in healthcare (Morrissey and Rivers, 1998).

School education in relation to sexual orientation is practically non-existent in many schools surveyed in America (Rienzo et al, 1996). Furthermore, research in relation to homosexuality and healthcare continues to be marked with sensitive ethical issues (Platzer and James, 1997). At present, sexuality is an area where ignorance, prejudice and morality hold sway. This is illustrated by providing a brief twentieth century history surrounding homosexuality and healthcare.

A brief twentieth century history (based on Sayce 1995)

Prior to the Second World War, the professional medical literature viewed homosexuality as an illness and/or as a pathology caused by problems in early development. At this time, psychoanalytic themes suggested that male homosexuals equated the penis with their mother's breast milk; that the passive homosexual is trying to extinguish the race and that 'society is justified in it's violent feelings towards him ... and in taking steps against him' (Lewes, 1988).

In Germany during the 1930s, a systematic repression of homosexuality included re-educating gay men, and to a lesser degree lesbians, into heterosexuality using psychological approaches; such re-education programmes were implemented at the Berlin Institute for Psychological Research and Psychotherapy. For example, in 1936, of the 50 000 men convicted of homosexuality, approximately 5000 were sent to concentration camps; how survivors dealt with their experiences is largely unknown (Grau, 1995). Some accounts are available eg. one gay survivor wrote a book about his experiences (Heger, 1980).

During the immediate post-war period, negative attitudes and oppressive practices continued. This is reflected in the fact that during 1951 lobotomy was used extensively to treat homosexuality in the US. Hospitalisation and other treatments, such as aversion therapy, remained common throughout the 1960s and beyond. By the end of the fifties, however, a more liberal approach began to emerge in the medical and psychological literature. In 1957, Evelyn Hooker published research showing that gay men could not be distinguished from heterosexual men on the basis of psychological tests, such as Rorschach ink blot tests. Gay men were within the normal psychological range. Her research was met with ridicule and disbelief by many mental health professionals. Further research lent support to Hooker's view, showing that there was no greater pathology or immaturity in lesbians than in other women (Sayce, 1995).

The late fifties and sixties marked a change in attitudes toward homosexuality. At the end of the fifties, homosexual relations in private between men over 21 were decriminalised in England following *The Wolfenden Report*. A decade later in 1969, saw the birth of gay liberation following rioting in response to a police raid on the Stonewall gay bar in New York. Two years later in 1971, The Gay Liberation Front (GLF) in the UK published its manifesto, which included 'psychiatry' on gay peoples' list of oppressors.

Demonstrations included jeering at psychiatrists in Harley Street. Gay and women's rights campaigners argued for declassifying homosexuality as a mental illness, drawing on Dr Hooker's research (Hooker, 1957) and in 1973 the American Psychiatric Association declassified homosexuality as a mental illness, but replaced it by ego-dystonic homosexuality. This disorder was to be diagnosed when people had confusions or disturbance about their sexual orientation (Sayce, 1995). The World Health Organization did not declassify homosexuality as a mental disorder until 1992. It was still possible to be gay and seen as mentally ill simply on that basis.

During the 1970s, professional and medical literature lagged behind the decision that homosexuality *per se* was not a mental illness. The British Medical Journal carried an article in 1975 discussing the potential for different treatments of homosexuality: for example, hormonal treatments; 'Great success has been claimed in treating homosexual men with stilboestrol or stilboestrol implant', therapy to deflect men from 'acting out illegally'; ie. publicly gay behaviour, and therapy to mobilise the heterosexual elements which are always present' (Williams, 1975).

There were many developments in the 1980s in and out of parliament. The parliament of 1982 debated a 'gay amendment' to the Bill which became the Mental Health Act (1983). The amendment would have given gay partners the same rights as heterosexuals to act as 'nearest relative' under the Act. The amendment was defeated. Self-help was set up by and for people infected or affected by HIV/AIDS. Much of the activity was done by gay men; major fund-raising activities by organisations like Cruisaid; birth of organisations, such as the Terence Higgins Trust, Body Positive and London Lighthouse pioneered the work of AIDS and addressed the emotional needs of gay men; development of lesbian information services and lesbian and gay counselling and therapy organisations like PACE.

Many other organisations developed. These included SHAKTI (South Asian) for ethnic minorities communities and the NAZ project which provides services and education around HIV/AIDS (Acquired

Immunodeficiency Syndrome), both organisations being based in London. In 1984, the European parliament adopted the Squarcialupi Report (Sayce, 1995), recommending equal rights for lesbians and gay men, including rejection of the classification of homosexuality as a mental illness.

Later, in 1986, the Greater London Council (GLC) called for an end to shock, drug or behavioural therapy to cure homosexuality and lesbianism. Much feeling was generated in the UK both in and outside the gay and lesbian community in relation to clause 28. Finally in 1988 Section 28 of the Local Government Act made it illegal for local authorities to promote homosexuality, which left authorities cautious about funding lesbian or gay support services. The Royal College of Nursing set up a working party to look at the nursing needs of lesbians and gay men

In the nineties, there is still much to be done to dispel myths and prejudices surrounding homosexuality. The British Psychological Society (BPS) in 1991 turned down the proposal for a lesbian section. Executive Secretary, Chris Newman, said that accepting such a section would mean the BPS was 'giving a public signal that it endorses behaviour which, by the biblical standards they personally seek to follow, is incompatible with their own standards of morality' (Holder, 1993). The Vatican put out a statement in 1992 describing homosexuality as an 'objective disorder' (Sayce, 1995).

The Department of Health (DoH, 1993) published Health of the Nation Key Area Handbook: Mental Illness, which includes reference to difficulties experienced by lesbians and gay men in accessing services. This is probably the first reference to lesbian and gay mental health issues in DoH policy. A DoH leaflet outlines that those at risk of suicide include people 'whose sexual orientation brings them into conflict with their family or others'. The UK government decided to strike homosexuality off its central computer list of mental disorders (DoH, 1993). There was also growing academic and media debate about the supposed 'gay gene' (D'Alessio, 1996). To some, this confirmed homosexuality as a disorder which could ultimately be reduced by genetic engineering; to others it meant that being homosexual was biologically determined and not a matter of choice.

There was a growing concern and a real attempt to equalise the age of consent for homosexual and heterosexual individuals. However, a recent attempt in 1994 failed to equalise the age of consent despite support from some mental health organisations including MIND and the Royal College of Psychiatrists. Twenty-two out of 28 countries in the Council of Europe now have an equal age of consent. Britain is the only country in NATO, with the exception of Turkey that still has a blanket ban on lesbians and gay men serving in the army. The 1994

Government Mental Health Nursing Review, *Working in Partnership*, states that gay or bisexual men or women should be treated sensitively (HMSO, 1994). Recently, Stonewall Immigration Group has successfully supported a number of cases in the courts and Jack Straw, the new Home Secretary, has said that immigration policy will be reviewed and same-sex couples will be recognised. The Inland Revenue has also said that pension schemes can recognise same-sex couples, although many schemes, particularly in the public sector, do not do so.

However, old prejudices die hard and in 1995 Professor Charles Socarides, an American psychoanalyst, was invited to give the annual lecture at the Association for Psychoanalytic Psychotherapy in London. He was well-known for campaigning before 1973 to keep homosexuality classified as a mental disorder and for his view that being gay is a developmental disorder. The talk was cancelled following protests. In the same year the Mental Health Foundation funded two projects focusing on lesbian and gay mental health issues: LYSIS (Lesbian Information Service) and 42nd Street in Manchester. In the late nineties Stonewall stepped up pressure in relation to equality for gay, lesbian and bisexual individuals (Stonewall, 1997). In 1996, gay marriages in Hawaii challenged the American legal system to promote equality in the constitution.

Amnesty International (1997) released a report that detailed the persecution of gays across the Third World. 'Social cleansing' by the Latin American death squads has resulted in the murders of hundreds of gay men in Brazil, Columbia and Mexico. 'Repulsive' homosexuals offend against 'the laws of nature', said President Robert Mugabe of Zimbabwe. They 'subvert the foundations of correct society', ruled the Nicaraguan Supreme Court. Terry Dicks, a prominent conservative MP in the UK, suggested that gays need 'a spray to stop them, or better still a red hot poker to make sure they would never do it again' (Cohen, 1997). Finally, in 1997–98 it is announced that there will be a 7% increase in the HIV treatment and care budget in the UK. Senior AIDS clinicians warn that the extra £14 million will not meet the growing bill for combination therapy and there are growing demands from the AIDS sector to spend carefully, define standards of care, become more equitable and efficient with less duplication of services, particularly in London (McKerrow and Edge, 1997).

Law

In the UK, a man can have sex lawfully with a woman of 16 years of age, but not with a man until 18 years of age. Lesbian sex has never been illegal in Britain, however, the age of consent is also 16-years-old. At present there is no legal redress for dismissal from work on the grounds of sexual orientation and discrimination is often the result (Greasley, 1986; Davies and Neal, 1996).

In America, private consensual sexual activities between adults of the same sex are criminal offences in 29 states (Carlson, 1990). Since 1982, the policy of the US Department of Defence has been that homosexuality is incompatible with military service. In January 1993 President Clinton announced his intention to reverse the military's ban and called for how best to implement a new, non-discriminatory policy (Herek, 1993). However, legislation has yet to follow. There is a multitude of challenges for same-sex relationships in legal terms to establish equal rights. Discrimination is a major obstacle. This is particularly true in employment, human rights, immigration, child custody, healthcare and insurance. Inequitable laws reinforce stereotypes and discrimination. It is clear that human rights and legal rights are not always equivalent but Paul Sieghart has made a great contribution to promoting human rights for people affected by AIDS in the UK (Sieghart, 1989). However, ignorance and prejudice are often present. One legal example is given below. A solicitor who specialises in lesbian custody cases noted the prurient obsession in the courts with sex:

> *'I've never had the case where a lesbian mother hasn't been asked in detail about her sex life.'* She recalls questions, such as *'Will you have sex in front of the children?' 'Do you make a noise when you have sex? Do you use appliances?'* (The witness reportedly replied: *'We've got a Hoover.'*)
>
> (Reported by Helen Garlick, *Guardian* 5/12/90 cited in Campion, 1995).

Religion and homosexuality

Perhaps being lesbian or gay has less to do with how you have sex, or even if you have sex at all, but rather with something else. Ram Dass (1994) suggests that sexuality has a real spiritual dimension, connected with identity and living meaningful lives. However, the impact of organised Christian religions on the spiritual well-being of lesbian, gay men and bisexual men and women has generally been sadly negative at best and frequently extremely destructive (Lynch, 1996). Based on more recent interpretations of scriptures, some scholars suggest that homosexuality is not a sin (Martin, 1984). According to Ram Dass, desire creates suffering and keeps our innermost selves from finding life's ultimate fulfilment: the state of being at one with God. Ram Dass suggests that whether you are gay, lesbian, bisexual or heterosexual makes no difference. He, himself, is gay and was a Professor of Harvard University between 1958 and 1963.

Unlike some small sections of eastern philosophy, mainstream religious churches do not accept or affirm homosexuality and lesbianism in terms of lifestyle or spirituality. From biblical, Islamic and Jewish fundamentalism to Roman Catholic dogmatism, lesbian, gay and bisexual people have been ostracised and persecuted (Lynch, 1996). Prophet Mohammed's view was that 'Allah has cursed him who indulges in this evil act of the people of Lut' (Haddith An Nasa'i, quoted in Thompson, 1994). Religion has been and is the most important negative force in shaping western attitudes and beliefs about sexuality (Lynch, 1996). The Society of Friends or Quakers are the only religious group which have publicly accepted homosexuality.

Generally, the needs of lesbian and gay men are not catered for in any of the Christian churches rituals or services. More recent challenges have been in relation to same-sex marriage and funerals which frequently neglect the partner (Wertheimer, 1987). At best, gays, lesbians and bisexuals are tolerated within a 'Love the sinner — hate the sin' framework. 'Homosexuals are disordered in their nature and evil in their love' (Cardinal Ratzinger, 1986). Many eastern religions seem similarly intolerant. However, individual ministers and laypersons have advocated for gay rights. Recently more pro gay religious organisations have been formed, such as Dignity for Gay Catholics, the Gay and Lesbian Christian group, and Integrity, for gay Episcopalians. Furthermore, there have been positive position statements made on homosexuality from the Episcopalians, Unitarians and Lutherans.

Homosexuality and healthcare

Health professionals

Medicine, psychology, psychiatry and psychoanalysis all have played, and in some respects continue to play, an instrumental part in creating and reinforcing negative and pathologising labels of many individuals who are gay, lesbian or bisexual. Sexuality has been described as the uninvited guest in the nurse-patient relationship (Savage, 1989). If this is so perhaps issues to do with lesbian, gay and bisexual clients have yet to be addressed by healthcare workers, such as nurses and doctors.

It has been pointed out that clinical information addressing the health needs of lesbians, gay and bisexual individuals was non-existent in medical and nursing texts and journals until the mid 1970s, (Carlson, 1990). This is no surprise given that such texts often lag behind current public opinion (Sayce, 1995).

The health needs of gay, lesbian and bisexual individuals can no longer be ignored given the persistent challenges from gay and lesbian organisations and the increase in research, public awareness and clinical information (Sieghart, 1989; Irwin, 1992; Platzer, 1993; Eliason, 1993; RCN, 1994; Morrissey, 1996; Rivers, 1996; Eliason, 1996). However, there is also a need to develop education and policies in practice (Sayce, 1995; RCN, 1994; Morrissey and Rivers, 1998).

Jackson (1995) has argued that introductory text books, while advocating objectivity and neutrality, often repathologise 'that which has been de-pathologised for twenty years' betraying the stereotypic attitudes and beliefs of the authors. Indeed, it would seem that, despite a general increase in our awareness of the existence of lesbians, gay men and bisexual men and women, homosexuality continues to be viewed as a perversion and little has been done to dispel this point of view (Davies and Neal, 1996). More generally, however, concerns have been raised with respect to the level of primary care offered to lesbians and gay men when they visit their local general practice or medical centre. Several recent reports have argued that, in the case of lesbian and bisexual women, the presumption of heterosexuality by clinicians has implications for the successful detection and treatment of a range of health-related issues including HIV infection, cancer screening, sexually-transmitted diseases, alcohol abuse, depression and domestic violence (see for example Rankow, 1995; Roberts and Sorensen, 1995; White and Levinson, 1995).

In the nursing literature, patients' rights, holistic care and high standards of care are vehemently upheld. In reality, only 'superficial lip service is paid to the acceptance of others as individuals with the freedom to choose how they live and the manner of their relationships' (Faugier and Wright, 1990). In the absence of a progressive educational philosophy which incorporates an affirmative approach to discussing homosexuality, stereotypic and stigmatic attitudes may well interfere both directly and indirectly with the care provided by health professionals (Scherer et al, 1991; Morrissey and Rivers, 1998). Platzer (1993) points out that there is evidence that doctors and nurses are prejudiced and fearful of lesbians and gay men. The emergence of HIV/AIDS has only served to reinforce such 'fear and loathing' expressed to a range of patients' groups associated with their illnesses (Green and Platt, 1997). Another prevailing belief is that family life and relationships for lesbians and gay men are somehow less important and less serious than heterosexual attachments.

Sometimes wrong assumptions are made, and clients may be fearful of disclosing their sexual orientation to a healthcare worker in case confidentiality is breached (Johnson et al, 1984). Furthermore, there can be prejudice when a gay man, lesbian or bisexual person becomes a patient (Irwin, 1992; Platzer, 1993; Morrissey, 1996).

Tierney (1995) suggests that, even though training is given, negative attitudes about gay and lesbian clients still prevail.

Homophobia results in stigma towards individuals who are attracted to and form loving same-sex relationships. In all disciplines such stigma and homophobia remain in relation to medicine, (Rose, 1994), nursing care (Tierney, 1995; Smith, 1993), psychotherapy (Davies and Neal, 1996), mental health services (Sayce, 1995), attitudes of practitioners to clients in their care (Morrissey, 1996; Rose, 1994) and nurse education (Morrissey and Rivers, 1998).

In a study on attitudes and homophobia among psychiatric nurses, Smith (1993) found that the majority of respondents (77%) indicated either moderate (57%) or severe homophobia (20%). It is suggested that while many nurses may have a cognitive acceptance of gays and lesbians, they continue to have deeply ingrained negative feelings towards them. In their study of 5000 practising nurses, Kelly *et al*, (1988) found that their sample reacted more negatively towards patients with HIV/AIDS than those with leukaemia, and that 'a very similar pattern of stigma was found for portrayals of individuals identified as homosexual, regardless of their illness'. The maintenance of social prejudices and stereotypes can have a significant effect upon the nature and effectiveness of the healthcare provided.

Traditional healthcare still has a heterosexual bias. The reality is that many healthcare providers may be unaware of gay, lesbian or bisexual individuals in their patient population. An example is found on nearly every health history form, 'Are you married?' Even though many same-sex couples are often in committed monogamous relationships, sometimes with children, there is no category that acknowledges the relationship. 'Single' denies that very important relationship and 'flat mate' minimises the relationship (Eliason, 1993). However, next-of-kin poses a more complex problem if healthcare providers only recognise heterosexual relationships or biological relations.

Currently, lesbian and gay partners have few (if any) rights in deciding the treatment or funeral arrangements for their dead partner and, because we continue to perceive 'next-of-kin' to mean husband/wife or nearest living relative, same-sex life partners are often left isolated and their wishes ignored by those responsible for dispensing care. This is sometimes further complicated by family conflict with partners.

'Harty cuts live-in pal out of will', highlights a problem all too common among gay men and lesbians that, at the death of a lover, the surviving partner is allowed no role in what comes next. Harty's lover, according to the report, has had to leave the house that they shared. Others have been denied access to their lover's body, have not been allowed to take part in the funeral arrangement and, in some cases have not been notified of the death. Lack of societal acknowledgement can inhibit, delay, prolong or completely supress the vital components of grief work, predisposing the individual to an abnormal grief reaction (Jones, 1989).

Due to such heterosexual bias, there may be non-acceptance of gays, the societal norm resulting in homophobia. Blumenfield (1992) suggests that the term 'homophobia' should be replaced by the term 'heterosexism' because homophobia fails to convey the true and complete extent of oppression based on sexual orientation.

Lesbian and gay individuals themselves may also have negative beliefs about their own sexuality that may result in a self-hatred which is related to one's own sexual identity (Gonsiorek and Rudolph, 1991). Heterosexism is defined as the belief that heterosexuality is, or should be, the only acceptable sexual orientation, while homophobia involves the fear and hatred of those who are sexually attracted to and love those of the same sex (Blumenfield, 1992).

This is often presented in overt but sometimes subtle ways in healthcare, placing 'high risk stickers' on everything from TPR charts to the drip chambers of sets for intravenous fluids. Patients have been avoided, ridiculed and exposed to an avalanche of negative and disapproving non-verbal behaviours (Irwin, 1992).

It may well be that some gay patients do not care what doctors and nurses think of them or their chosen lifestyle, but as Faugier and Wright (1990) state, 'All patients have the right to anticipate respect and regard from those entrusted with their care'. Pogoncheff (1979) described the 'care' a lesbian patient in one American hospital experienced and concludes: 'We had denied her basic comfort measures and treated her in a mechanical and businesslike way when we did offer physical care. We'd stereotyped her and kept her at a distance emotionally. We had, in fact, promoted instability in a patient' (Pogoncheff, 1979). Even if individual doctors and nurses are not prejudiced and seek to provide non-judgmental care regardless of sexual orientation, they may inadvertently be affected by commonly held beliefs and stereotypes.

It is often assumed, for example, that lesbians and gay men do not have and do not want to have children. This is clearly untrue as many lesbians and gay men do have children either from previous heterosexual relationships, or after they have 'come out'. Many plan to have children as lesbians or gay men. Lack of awareness of this can lead to inappropriate consideration of fertility during medical treatment, and insensitive care when future fertility is uncertain (Platzer, 1993).

Many health professionals who are themselves lesbian, gay or bisexual continue to remain invisible because of homophobia. Many individuals, such as doctors may have been negatively affected by homophobic prejudice when their sexual orientation was revealed (Rose, 1994). Homophobia predates AIDS, but AIDS fosters further prejudice and homophobia (Tierney, 1995). Many gay men have reservations about approaching traditional healthcare services due to fear of stigma and prejudice (Taylor and Robertson, 1994).

Although there may be a move to accommodate the needs of lesbian women, gay men and bisexual individuals, health professionals should not be complacent. In practice, all health professionals need to be involved in education in order to examine their feelings, values, and knowledge towards homosexuality to improve and inform care (Morrissey and Rivers, 1998).

If healthcare is to be genuinely available to all clients, irrespective of sexuality or sexual identity, it is essential that such issues are addressed in the education and training of nurses, doctors and other health professionals. Priority needs to be placed on clear healthcare policies which uphold and protect the rights of all clients. The positive contribution made to society by lesbian, gay or bisexual people is now recognised. Is it not time for healthcare professionals to embrace cultural diversity, instead of maintaining negative and prejudicial attitudes towards men and women simply because of their sexual orientation?

References

American Psychiatric Association (1973) cited in: Sayce L (1995) *Breaking the Link between Homosexuality and Mental Illness. An Unfinished History*. MIND, London

Barbone S, Rice L (1994) Coming out, being out, and acts of virtue. Gay ethics: Controversies in outing, civil rights, and sexual science. *J Homosex* **27**(3–4): 91–110

Batcup D, Thomas B (1994) Mixing the genders, an ethical dilemma: How nursing has dealt with sexuality and gender. *Nurs Ethics* **1**(1) 43–52

Blumenfield WT (1992) *Homophobia: How We All Pay the Price*. Beacon, Boston

Boswell J (1996) *The Marriage of Likeness: Same-Sex Unions in Pre-Modern Europe*. Fontana Press, London

Bullough V (1979) *Homosexuality: A History*. New York Meridian Books/New American Library, New York

Campion M (1995) *Who's Fit to be a Parent?* Routledge, London

Carlson BN (1990) Gay and lesbian lifestyles. Cited in: Fogel CI, Lauver D. *Sexual Health Promotion*. WB Saunders, Philadelphia: 117–32

Chekola M (1994) Outing, truth-telling, and the shame of the closet. Gay ethics: Controversies in outing, civil rights and sexual science. *J Homosex* **27**(3–4): 67–90

Clift S, Kanabus A, Callister C, Forrest S (1996) *Condoms, Pills and Other Useful Things*. Avert, Horsham:

Clift S, Kanabus A, Callister C, Forrest S (1997) *Sexual Feelings and Relationships*. Avert, Horsham:

Cohen N (1997) Two-faced Tories face both ways on gay rights. *The Observer* 23 February: 20

Davies D, Neal C (1996) Pink Therapy: A Guide for Counsellors Working with Lesbian, Gay and Bisexual Clients. Open University Press, Buckingham

D'Alessio V (1996) Born to be gay. *New Scientist* September: 32–5

Dejowski EF (1992) Public endorsement on restrictions of three aspects of free expression by homosexuals: Socio-demographic and trends analysis 1973–1988. *J Homosex* **23**(4): 1–18

Department of Health (1993) *Health of The Nation Key Area Handbook: Mental Illness*. HMSO, London

Eliason MJ (1993) Cultural diversity in nursing care: the lesbian, gay or bisexual client. *J Transcult Nurs* **5**(1): 14–20

Eliason MJ (1996) Institutional barriers to healthcare for lesbian, gay and bisexual persons. *NLN Publications* 14-6762: (273P).

Epting FR, Raskin JD, Burke TB (1994) Who is homosexual? A critique of the heterosexual-homosexual distinction. Special Theme: Body and soul. *Humanist Psychol* **22**(3): 353–70

Faugier J, Wright S (1990) Homophobia, stigma, and AIDS: an issue for all healthcare workers. *Nurs Practice* **3**(2): 27–8

Fogel CI, Lauver D (1990) *Sexual Health Promotion*. WB Saunders, Philadelphia

Forrest S, Biddle G, Clift S (1997) Talking About Homosexuality in the Secondary School. Avert, Horsham

Frankham J, Kanabuss A (1996) *Young Gay Men Talking*. Avert, Horsham

Gallop Report (1982) cited In: Sayce L (1995) *Breaking the Link Between Homosexuality and Mental Illness. An Unfinished History*. MIND, London

GLC (1986) *Tackling Heterosexism*. GLC, London

Gonsiorek JC, Rudolph JR (1991) Homosexual identity: coming out and other developmental events. In: Gonsiorek GC, Weinrich JD, eds. *Homosexuality: Research Implications for Public Policy*. Sage Publications, Newbury Park, CA

Grau G (1995) *The Hidden Holocaust: Gay and Lesbian Persecution in Germany 1935–45*. Cassell, London

Greasley P (1986) *Gay Men at Work*. Lesbian and Gay Employment Rights, London

Green G, Platt S (1997) Fear and loathing in healthcare settings reported by people with HIV. *Sociol Health Illness* **19**(N01): 70–92

Harry J (1993) Being out: A general model. *J Homosex* **26**(1): 25–39

Heger H (1980) *The Men with the Pink Triangle*. Gay Mens Press, London

Herek GM (1993) Sexual orientation and military service. A social science perspective. *Am Psychol* **48**(5) 538–49

Holder D (1993) Should lesbians be sectioned? *Gardian* **6 Jan**: 9

Hooker EA (1957) The adjustment of the male overt homosexual. *J Protect Techniq* **21**: 17–31

Irwin R (1992) Critical re-evaluation can overcome discrimination: Providing equal standards of care for homosexual patients. *Prof Nurse* **April**: 435–8

Jackson D (1995) Nursing texts and lesbian contexts: lesbian imagery in the nursing literature. *Aus J Adv Nurs* **13**(1): 25–31

Johnson SR, Palermo JL (1984) Gynaecological care for the lesbian. *Clin Obstet Gynaecol* **27**(3): 724–31

Jones A (1989) Managing the invisible grief. *Sen Nurse* **9**(5): 26–7

Joseph H (1993) Being out: A general model. *J Homosex* **26**(1): 25–39

Kelly JA, St Lawrence JS, Hood HV, Smith S Jr, Cook D (1988) Nurse attitudes towards AIDS. *J Cont Educ* **19**(2): 78–83

Kleis BN, Lock J (1995) The public discussion of homosexuality. *J Am Acad Child Adolesc Psychiatry* **34**(1): 6

Lewes K (1988) *The Psychoanalytic Theory of Male Homosexuality*. Simon and Schuster, New York

(Lucian) Affairs of the Heart (1996) Edited and translated by Macleod, MD in (1967). Cited in: Boswell J *The Marriage of Likeness: Same Sex Unions in Pre-Modern Europe*. Fontana Press, London

Lynch B (1996) Religious and spirituality conflicts. In: Davies D, Neal C, eds. *Pink Therapy: A Guide for Counsellors Working with Lesbian, Gay and Bisexual Clients*. Open University Press, Buckingham, PA

Magee M, Miller DC (1994) Psychoanalysis and women's experiences of 'coming out': The necessity of becoming a 'bee charmer'. *J Acad Psychoanal* **22**(3): 481–504

Martin AD (1984) The perennial Canaanites: the sin of homosexuality. *Rev Gen Seman* **41**: 340–61

Martin AD, Hetrick ES (1988) The Stigmatisation of the gay and lesbian adolescent: In Ross MW, ed. *The Treatment of Homosexuals with Mental Health Disorders*. Harrington Park Press, New York

Mason A, Watson M (1997) *Equality 2000*. Stonewall, London

McKerrow G, Edge S (1997) Disarray on Dorrell cash signals conflict to come. *Positive Nation.* **14**: 13

Meyer JK (1985) Ego-dystonic homosexuality. In: Kaplan H, Sadock B, eds. *Comprehensive Textbook of Psychiatry IV.* Williams and Wilkins, Baltimore

Millard J (1995) Suicide and suicide attempts in the lesbian and gay community. *Aust N Z J Ment Health Nurs* **4**(4): 181–9

Morrissey M (1996) Attitudes of practitioners to lesbian, gay and bisexual clients. *Br J Nurs* **5**(16): 980–2

Morrissey M, Rivers I (1998) Applying the Mims-Swenson Sexual Health Model to nurse education: Offering an alternative focus on sexuality and healthcare. *Nurse Educ Today* **18**: 488–95

Morrow DF (1993) Social work with gay and lesbian adolescents. *Soc Work* **38**(6): 655–9

Nelson JA (1997) Gay lesbian and bisexual adolescents providing esteem-enhancing care to a battered population. Nurse practitioner. *Am J Prim Healthcare* **22**(2): 94–9

Platzer H (1993) Nursing care for gay and lesbian patients. *Nurs Stand* **7**(17): 35–7

Platzer H, James T (1997) Methodological difficulties conducting sensitive research on lesbians and gay men's experience of nursing care. *J Adv Nurs* **25**(3): 626–33

Pogoncheff E (1979) The gay patient. *Reg Nurse* **April**: 46–52

Ram Dass (1994) A life beyond labels. In: Thompson M, ed. *Gay Soul.* Harper Collins, San Francisco

Rankow EJ (1995) Lesbian health issues for the primary care provider. *J Fam Pract* **40**(5): 486–96

Ratzinger J (1986) On pastoral care of homosexual people. *Congregation for the Doctrine of the Faith.* Vatican City, on Halloween, 31 October.

Report of the Mental Health Nursing Review (1994) *Working in Partnerships.* HMSO, London

Rienzo BA, Button J, Wald KD (1996) The politics of school-based programs which address sexual orientation. *J School Health* **66**(1): 33–40

Rivers I (1996) The victimisation of lesbian, gay and bisexual youth. Paper presented at the *Research on Lesbian, Gay and Bisexual Youths: Implications for Developmental Intervention Conference.* The Pennsylvania State University, USA, 7–9 June.

Roberts SJ, Sorensen L (1995) Lesbian healthcare: a review and recommendations for health promotion in primary care settings. *Nurse Practitioner* **20**(6): 42–7

Rose L (1994) Homophobia among doctors. *Br Med J* **308**: 586–7

Rotheram B, Jane M, Fernandez I (1995) Sexual orientation and development challenges experienced by gay and lesbian youths. *Suicide Life Threat Behav* **25**(Suppl): 26–34

Royal College of Nursing (1994) *The Nursing Care of Lesbians and Gay Men: An RCN Statement*. RCN, London

Savage J (1989) Sexuality: an uninvited guest. *Nurs Times* **85**(5): 25–8

Sayce L (1995) *Breaking the Link Between Homosexuality and Mental Illness. An Unfinished History*. MIND, London

Scherer YK, Wu YW, Haughey BP (1991) AIDS and homophobia among nurses. *J Homosexual* **21**: 17–27

Sell RL, Wells JA, Valleron A-J, Will A, Cohen M, Umbel K (1990) Homosexual and bisexual behaviour in the United States, the United Kingdom and France. Paper presented at *the Sixth International Conference on AIDS*. San Francisco

Sieghart P (1989) *AIDS and Human Rights: A UK Perspective*. British Medical Association Foundation for AIDS, London

Smith GB (1993) The nursing care challenges of homosexual psychiatric patients. *J Psychosoc Nurs* **30**: 15–21

Socarides C (1995) You decide: should this man be gagged? *Daily Mail* **27 April**: 16–17

Taylor I, Robertson A (1994) The health needs of gay men: a discussion of the literature and implications for nursing. *J Adv Nurs* 20(3): 560–6

Thompson M (1994) *Gay Soul*. Harper Collins, San Francisco

Thompson R (1993) *Religion, Ethnicity, Sex Education: Exploring the Issues*. National Children's Bureau, London

Tierney AJ (1995) HIV/AIDS knowledge, attitudes and education of nurses: a review of research. *J Clin Nurs* **4**(1): 13–21

Walters AS, Phillips CP (1994) An activity for homosexuality education. *J Sex Educ Ther* **20**(3): 198–203

Weinrich JD, Williams WL (1991) Strange customs, familiar lives: homosexualities in other cultures. In: Gonsiorek GC, Weinrich JD, eds. *Homosexuality: Research Implications for Public Policy*. Sage Publications, Newbury Park

Wertheimer A (1987) Mourning in secret. *New Soc* **17 April**: 8–9

White JC, Levinson W (1995) What a primary care physician needs to know. *West J Med* **162**(5): 463–6

Williams AH (1975) Problems of homosexuality. *Br Med J* **3**(5980): 426–8

World Health Organization (1992) *International Statistical Classification of Diseases and Related Health Problems* (ICD) Tenth Revision. WHO, Geneva

6
Sexuality and the child

Cherry Bennett

Give me a child until he is seven and I will give you the man.

(attributed to the Jesuits)

This quote epitomises for many the fact that what children learn in their early years will have an effect on them in adulthood. To an increasing extent, this can be seen in terms of health with evidence, for example, that lifelong eating patterns established during childhood may have marked implications for future health, particularly with regard to coronary heart disease (Department of Health, 1994).

Health, however, encompasses more than merely physical aspects. The issue of sexual health has been somewhat ignored and yet, arguably, it is a vital component of health and well-being and an important aspect to be considered in children if they are to reach their full potential. Curtis *et al* (1995) suggest that the nature of British society is hypocritical and forms a barrier to sexual health promotion. Curtis *et al* continue by stating that the media exploits sexuality and sex through film, television, literature and music, yet sex is viewed as a private and hidden affair, if not a little embarrassing, especially to talk about on a personal level.

It can be suggested that the government has taken a step forward in this arena by identifying sexual health as one of five key areas in the strategy for the *Health of the Nation* (Department of Health, 1992). The objectives are:

- to reduce the incidence of HIV infection
- to reduce the incidence of other sexually-transmitted diseases (STD)
- to strengthen monitoring and surveillance
- to provide effective services for diagnosis and treatment of HIV and other STDs
- to reduce the number of unwanted pregnancies
- to ensure the provision of effective family planning services for those people who want them.

The strategy is based on an illness model which aims to reduce mortality and morbidity whereas it could be considered more appropriate to view sexual health in terms of interventions which improve a person's physical or sexual well-being.

Learning about sexuality

Children learn through various means and from a variety of sources. The way children learn about sexuality and sexual health stems predominantly from the family. There are, of course, biological differences but as Webb (1985) believes, how we view ourselves and how others react to us as sexual beings is something we learn. From the moment a baby is born, its biological sex will influence the way it will be treated by its parents, perhaps unconsciously. This is a result of what the parents have learned and thus the pattern of role differentiation between sexes continues against the background of other social structures, such as cultural definitions of gender and the sexual division of labour.

Within western cultures, children learn about sex role behaviour as early as two years of age when both dressing and play is based on what they have already learned (Oakley, 1972; cited in Webb, 1985). The type of toys given will often differ between boys and girls and in this way they are likely to play with objects which symbolise later gender roles. However, when a choice of different gender type toys are available, girls will play with the more masculine type of toy, but boys are less likely to play with the feminine type toys.

Boys are generally expected to be more aggressive than girls and engage in boisterous play. Indeed aggression is socially valued culturally in males and, as such, certain behaviour is more readily accepted in boys than in girls. Such differentiation also occurs in relation to sexuality, certainly as the child grows and develops. In many ways young people are expected to behave in a more sexual manner; boys buy the latest after-shave to attract females almost before they have any facial hair and girls dress to be attractive to the opposite sex. Thus it can be seen that sex role stereotypes exist and are important to consider as older children may feel pressured to adopt them.

Current sociological changes may affect factors previously associated with specific gender roles that may in turn alter children's views. With increasing numbers of women employed outside the home, the more traditional role of women as housewives is being challenged and the view of the male as the 'breadwinner' is no longer the case for many families.

It would be difficult to write of how children learn about sexuality without mentioning the work of different theorists, particularly Piaget and Freud. However, it is not the intention to write at any great length about their work, but the following overview considers the perspectives in which children learn.

Piaget (1951; cited in Rutter, 1971) dominated the field of cognitive development wherein he believed that children pass through three stages to adolescence with the fundamental view that the cognitive stage of development was the most important factor in determining an individual's behaviour and attitude. Each of the three stages, sensory-motor, concrete and operational are related to children's chronological age and therefore each stage represented development within a particular age range.

On the other hand, Freud (1923; cited in Rutter, 1971), a psychoanalyst, described psychosexual stages of development which he suggested occurred at similar chronological ages to Piaget's stages of cognitive development. Freud's theories were based on the anatomical distinctions between the sexes and maintained that it was this which led to the development of two different personalities.

According to Freud, all children early on in life are unaware of differences between males and females and that sexual pleasure is gained from many body parts such as the mouth, anus and genitals. It is only later at around five years of age, suggests Freud, that children realise males and females are anatomically different. It is thus that the 'Oedipal phase' develops where girls feel inferior due to lack of a penis and a rivalry between mother and daughter builds in the relationship with the father. For a boy this Oedipal phase results in fantasies of a sexual nature with his mother and rivalry between son and father. Sexual pleasures for a boy are transferred to the penis.

Freud believes that by puberty this Oedipal complex is resolved and for both sexes different notions of sexuality have developed. For girls sexuality is a passive process, while for boys an active type of sexuality ensues (Webb, 1985).

Although much of Freud's thinking has formed the basis of sexual development, his work has been challenged and criticised. Children have developed concepts of femininity and masculinity earlier than Freud suggested. Different societies and their development of sexuality would also disprove aspects of his theories.

What is sexuality

It is easy to think that the term 'sexuality' relates to the physical activity of sex, but it should be considered in a much wider context. It is a powerful and emotive subject and cannot be easily defined, although many have tried. Perhaps consideration of the concept of sexuality is an easier task and Oijen and Charnock (1995) cite examples by Foucault (1979) and Gagnon and Simons (1973). Each had valuable contributions to make and aspects, such as relationships, culture and social interactions were used to describe the concept of sexuality. It should be remembered that sexuality will mean different things to different people and that views will change over time. The Victorian era was viewed publicly as one where chastity and repressed sexuality were the order of the day, to the point where even table legs were hidden. In reality, sexual excesses and promiscuity were common.

Sexuality is more than the physical, biological side of sex; it is not just the physical ability to reproduce, but is an integral part of humanity. Self-image and self-esteem are also facets which must be considered when interpretating sexuality. If, as nurses, it is the intention to cater for the needs of children, we must be clear about what those needs are, and an understanding of sexuality and all it comprises becomes crucial. If someone were to ask about a child's needs in terms of breathing, comprehension would be clear, but what if those needs were connected with sexuality, would comprehension follow?

Sexuality is a fundamental part of being human. It is more than our genital nature, reflecting our human character. It includes all those aspects that relate to being boy or girl, woman or man and is subject to lifelong, dynamic change. Again, sexuality is often regarded as an adult concept that has little to do with children. This is not, nor should it be the case. Sexuality is a normal part of human development and continues throughout the life cycle. It may be experienced differently during this cycle, but it must not be disregarded at certain stages as being unimportant, particularly in childhood.

In order for children to grow and develop with a healthy concept of sexuality, they must value themselves as a worthwhile human being. In doing so they will develop a positive self-image and high self-esteem. Pletsch *et al* (1991) are supportive of the view that a healthy conceptualisation of the self and self-image is an important foundation for functioning in later life. Farrand and Cox (1993) cite the works of Tax (1983) and Herold *et al* (1979) who considered that, in adolescents, there were 'positive relationships between self-esteem and positive health practices; adolescent girls with high self-esteem tended to be non-smokers and have more positive attitudes toward using birth control'. A favourable self-image is likely to affect children in other ways. They will be more confident in their own abilities, willing to voice opinions and be more accepting of criticism. Self-esteem should not be considered as a static concept, something we are born with. The effect of self-esteem on our behaviour is a dynamic interaction and may alter over time.

Although it can be suggested that family interactions and parenting styles may not be specific in terms of health behaviour, it is undoubtedly the case that the family environment forms the context in which health behaviours and perceptions are established.

Parents have an important role to play in the development of children's self-concept, as well as how they view sexuality. Children need to feel good about their bodies; bodily changes need to be explained and discussed in an open way so that the child is neither ashamed or embarrassed. Within some families this is not easy. Some parents feel unable to explain these bodily changes to their children. Birch (1992) suggests that a child's developing sexuality may pose a threat to the parents, especially if there are underlying marital problems. Allowing their child's individuality may be difficult for some parents and to this, already complex situation, may be added the fact that the mother or father may be jealous of their child's developing sexuality. On the other hand, it is possible that fathers, in particular, can be influential in a very positive way. A father who encourages his daughter not to become dependent on male approval for a sense of self-esteem will increase her feelings of independence and self-confidence. In this way she will be prepared to cope with criticism and rejection which may be encountered from other males and will contribute to her own sexual self-esteem. In terms of physical sexual development, there are few changes before puberty and although these changes usually occur over a four to five year period, timing for individual children varies considerably. It is, however, a time which often results in intense self-consciousness and is of psychological significance. Rutter (1971) cites examples indicating that boys are less confident, less popular and less assertive when they are late reaching puberty, but are talkative and attention-seeking. In today's society athletic ability is highly valued in most adolescent groups and it can, therefore, be seen how the above findings affects boys who have not attained the muscular physique associated with early puberty.

For many girls, early maturing does not appear to have the clear-cut advantages found in boys. In fact, it may be that very early maturing in girls can sometimes be associated with undue self-consciousness and anxiety. Attempts may be made to conceal breast development by wearing loose fitting clothes or altering posture. The onset of menstruation can also be viewed differently and cause varying reactions. If seen as a normal part of the developing process it will be approached calmly. However, if parents and friends act as though the girl needs sympathy, a negative reaction may result, growing up is resented and the ability to make a satisfactory feminine identification may be affected.

Thus, it can be seen that the age of puberty should not be dismissed lightly. Although, as already stated, most physical developmental changes occur at puberty, psychosexual development begins in infancy. Rutter (1971) cited in Friedrich *et al* (1991) reported a variety of sexualised behaviours in younger children which were viewed as 'normal". Such behaviours included erections in male infants, genital handling and masturbatory activity. A feature also common in children between 4 and 6 years was exhibitionistic and voyeuristic activities with other children and adults. Friedrich *et al* (1991) suggest that three to six years old is 'the developmental stage when children can be outrageously flirtatious and seductive, impersonating mannerisms of parents, older siblings, television actors or whoever'. Elementary age children progress through a stage where modesty and inhibitions are the focus. At an earlier age such children would openly undress in front of their parents, but as they approach the teenage years, bathroom privacy begins to be demanded and children are unlikely to discuss romantic aspects and 'boy/girlfriends' with adults.

Relationships with children of the opposite sex will also alter throughout childhood. Up to the age of approximately seven or eight years old, boys and girls play together. A phase then appears when children play predominantly with others of the same sex. Following this, at around puberty, social interaction with the opposite sex increases.

Thus it can be seen that throughout childhood and adolescence, both physical and psychosexual development takes place. As Friedrich *et al* (1991) state 'sexual behaviour of the child does not emerge in isolation'. It develops against a background of variables and the family is particularly influential in the formation of sexuality and sexual health.

Sexuality and child care

The argument for having specially trained nurses to look after children follows the belief that children are different from adults and have different needs. This can be said in relation to sexual health as well as physical and psychological aspects. Undeniably sexuality in children is different to that of adults, but what must be remembered is that it is different, not absent. Nurses working in a child care setting will be caring for children across an age span of 0 to 16 or 18 years. Although numerically this may not seem particularly great, in terms of development both physically and psychologically, it is considerable. It ranges from babies whose sexual health needs are minimal to adolescents whose sexual health needs may be paramount. This degree of variance requires flexibility in a nurse and, even more importantly, sensitivity to these very intimate needs.

Nursing has evolved over the years from a medical model basis to a profession capable of recognising the wider aspects of patient care and care delivery. Greater emphasis is now placed on the holistic care of patients, and as Webb (1985) suggests 'holistic care is much discussed'. Some eleven years on, it can be said that Webb's views still hold true, certainly in the child care field.

If sexuality is part of the totality of being human and the fundamental view of nursing is one of holism, how can it be that sexuality is not incorporated as vital component of care delivery? In reality, sexual health is a relatively new area for nurses to consider. Nursing has its roots based very firmly in tradition and external factors as well as factors within the profession continue to support the notion that anything to do with sexuality is a taboo subject.

Men do enter nursing but it remains a female-dominated profession. Most people's image of nurses are of women and throughout the socialisation process, this view is generally perpetuated. When men enter nursing, there is the implication that they are undertaking women's work and the view of them as 'real men' is often questioned. It is seen that women use their 'softer, feminine and maternal natures to care for the sick' (Webb, 1985). Men on the other hand disturb this social expectation and even when they do enter the profession, the different types of nursing in which they specialise is seen to follow particular routes. Men who enter child care nursing are relatively few in number and the same applies to health visiting and district nursing.

It is unfortunate that such stereotypical views persist, often based on inaccurate information and prejudice both of which are, nonetheless, powerful notions. In terms of sexual health, it can be argued that men have a particular place when discussing boys' sexual health needs. A youth may feel more comfortable discussing certain aspects of sexuality with someone of the same sex. Although changes are gradually taking place, issues concerning sexual health have frequently been ignored or covered inadequately within nurse education, and if this is the case, it is little wonder that sexual health needs are disregarded in practice.

For the majority of people open discussion of sexual health needs is not easy and many factors have led to this situation. Cultural political and social constraints are influential, but the socialisation of nurses themselves also pose barriers. For nurses working with children, many are not much older than those for whom they are caring, and it could be argued that they are in a position to discuss sexual health issues more openly. For some, this may indeed be the case, but for many, as a result of socialisation processes with respect to nursing and sexuality, it will be avoided. Rafferty (1995) believes that nurses commonly perceive their patients as being asexual because of the intimate nature of their work and as a result ignore an important aspect of the patient's well-being, namely the sexual aspects.

It could be said that British society is somewhat hypocritical towards sexual health matters. Young people may find it difficult to come to terms with developing the ability to control their own sexuality. The media exploits sexuality through music, literature, television and films and young people engaged in sexual activity are often portrayed as being promiscuous. Conversely, demands are made for sexual propriety with sex viewed as a private and hidden affair, discussion of which is an embarrassing topic. This then is the background against which children and those caring for them must proceed. Curtis *et al* (1995) suggests that 'denial of sexuality in childhood, the way in which children's sexual behaviour is viewed can promote openness about sexuality or covert guilt and shame from an early age'. It is therefore imperative that nurses caring for children acknowledge their own sexuality and the factors which have shaped it in order for them to address the health needs of others in an effective manner.

The way forward

The acceptance of children as having sexual health needs will not happen short-term. As with many other aspects of nursing, it will be a gradual process. There is little doubt that changes in the nursing care of children is now much more focussed on family-centred care. Just as the family were seen as fundamental so it can be said is children's sexual health. Increasingly the use of nursing models as a framework towards more holistic care has been a positive step with Roper *et al* (1980) identifying the expression of sexuality as one of the daily living activities. However, caution must be used to ensure that it is not raised as an issue inappropriately or as purely theoretical. Issues concerning sexual health have frequently been ignored or covered inadequately within nurse education and it is not surprising that sexual health needs are disregarded in practice. The subject of sexual health is difficult to broach and if both the child and the nurse are embarrassed, it is likely to be ignored. To minimise this, it is essential for sexual health to be discussed openly within the education of children in general and for the subject to become more overt within nurse education in order for nurses to develop confidence in increasing intervention within practice. This is necessary at both pre- and post-registration levels. Rafferty (1985) highlights the clinical learning environment as being a powerful culture and students are unlikely to incorporate sexual healthcare into their practice if they do not see qualified staff doing so.

Sexuality is related to gender and social issues and both should be included in nurses' education, and considered together with the biological aspects of sexuality. In order for nurses to gain knowledge and understanding of a patient's sexuality, they need to be aware of their own. It is necessary for them to consider their own attitudes and behaviour in order to attempt to provide non-judgmental care. When staff are knowledgeable about, and secure in their own sexuality, they are more comfortable in dealing with the sexual aspects of their work. This is not an easy task as many nurses who care for children are young themselves and still, to some extent, diffident about their own sexuality making discussion with someone younger or similar in age, embarrassing and difficult (Proctor and Swiniford, 1996).

If nurses feel that sexuality is a private matter then it is easy to ignore its relevance as an aspect of care. Children and adolescents do not discard their sexuality when they become ill or develop a chronic illness. On the contrary, sexual health needs could be even more important. It is imperative, therefore, for the issue to be addressed in order for children to receive the holistic care they need and deserve.

The inclusion of sexual health in children as a focus within the nurse education curriculum is a beginning, but it must not stand in isolation. Caring for children's sexual health cannot be undertaken in theory alone, it has to be incorporated into practice.

During the assessment stage, children's nurses need to give greater emphasis to the identification of sexual health needs of children with acute and chronic conditions. Children in hospital may well have a change in body image either visible or hidden and this should be considered. A detailed history may not be necessary but acknowledgement of sexual health needs must be made. For example, although a teenager may have had a long-term history of eczema, it does not mean that their body image or self-esteem remains constant. Confronting their image when placed in a hospital bay with two members of the opposite sex, but of a similar age, may make them feel less positive. This also raises the question of segregation. In adult wards males and females are generally nursed in separate bays yet children in their early teens are often in mixed sex bays. At what point should segregation be considered?

It is usually common practice for at least one parent to be in attendance during the assessment stage and this may cause difficulty in trying to determine sexual health needs. The child may be happier to discuss these at a later date when negotiation of care can take place. As with all aspects of history taking, privacy must be assured and the issue of confidentiality is an important consideration.

The Roper, Logan and Tierney model of nursing incorporates sexuality and, in many child care settings, care is planned using this model and, if used correctly, children's sexual health needs will be addressed.

Newton (1991) when looking at the model closely, suggests that as well as factors directly associated with problems relating to sexual organs or function, aspects of femininity and masculinity, the way the individual perceives him/herself and body image are all relevant and should also be considered.

Interestingly, the model also incorporates the opportunity to consider lifespan. However, from the author's experience, this part of the model is seldom used. Described in the model literature are eight developmental stages, the first four, namely prenatal, infancy, childhood and adolescence having particular relevance to those caring for children. In order to apply the model effectively in practice, use of the lifespan approach alongside the activities of living requires the nurse to be aware of the developmental stages of children.

Using a care study approach, Newton (1991) cites an example of how the nurse can consider the issue of sexuality in planning the care of a three-year-old boy needing eye surgery for correction of a squint. His normal routine was verified and noted. This included information that he was not 'modest or embarrassed about undressing or lavatory. Has not commented on appearance of squint' (Newton, 1991).

Such an example demonstrates clearly how and what aspects of sexual health can be identified in a relatively young child. It can be suggested that information of this nature should be obtained for all children in order to plan and deliver holistic care and that when using Roper, Logan and Tierney's model the activity of 'expressing sexuality' must not be discarded as irrelevant just because the patient is a child.

The education system has a role to play if children are to develop with a greater understanding and acceptance of their sexual health needs. Sex education often forms part of personal, social and health education in school, although to what degree and how it is taught varies considerably. Curtis *et al* (1995) identify the legal framework in England and Wales:

- in all state schools, the governing body must produce a written policy on sex education
- parents have a right to withdraw their children from sex education, where this falls outside the national curriculum
- at primary and secondary levels, some sexual and reproductive biology is taught in the national curriculum and is compulsory for all pupils. Parents cannot withdraw children from this
- at secondary level, schools must provide a wider programme of sex education, which goes beyond the national curriculum and must include HIV/AIDS and STDs

- at primary level, it is for the governors to decide whether or not to provide a wider programme of sex education. It is good practice to do so
- sex education must, as far as is reasonably practical, be taught in a manner that encourages due regard for moral considerations and the value of family life.

However, Stainland and Newell (1996) found much criticism of the system among pupils. It was felt that the information was not pitched correctly and delivered too late because the pupils are seen to be too young to talk about it. Indeed, there is the belief that the provision of knowledge may lead to increased promiscuity and early sexual experimentation, but Wellings *et al* (1995) point out 'more sex education does not mean more sex'.

Conclusion

This chapter has illustrated that sexuality is a very real component of the developing child and should be given due consideration alongside the physical, psychological and social development of the child. Although different to adults, children too have sexual health needs and this must be acknowledged in order to give effective healthcare to children of all ages. Recognising this and providing the opportunities for discussion of such needs in an open and trusting relationship can enhance the care given to children and their families.

An approach on a widespread scale may be required to facilitate this. Society in general must take a more open view in accepting sexuality as an integral part of the developing child. Children have the right to develop, as far as is possible, with a healthy self-image and respect for themselves. If they are able to discuss matters of sexuality comfortably at home and school they are more likely to accept their own sexuality.

In the interests of child health, nurses must be at the forefront in the facilitation of such an evolutionary process.

References

Birch D (1992) *Inner Worlds and Outer Challenges*. Youth Support Publications, London

Curtis H, Hoolaghan T, Jewitt C (1995) *Sexual Health Promotion in General Practice*. Radcliffe Medical Press, Oxford

Department of Health (1992) *The Health of the Nations*. HMSO, London

Department of Health (1994) *Report of Working Group on Weaning Diet of the Committee of Medical Aspects of Food Policy: Weaning and Weaning Diet*. HMSO, London

Farrand L, Cox C (1993) Determinants of positive health behaviour in middle childhood. *Nurs Res* **42**(4): 208–13

Foucault M (1979) *History of Sexuality*. Allen Lane, London

Freud S (1923) cited in Rutter M (1971) Normal psychosexual development. *J Child Psychol Psychiatry* **11**: 259–83

Friedrich W, Grambsch P, Broughton D, Koiper J, Beilke R (1991) Normative sexual behaviour in children. *Paediatrics* **88**(3) 456–64

Gagnon J, Simon W (1973) *Sexual Construct: The Social Sources of Human Sexuality*. Aldine Publishing, Chicago

McGurk H ed. (1992) *Childhood Social Development*. Erlbaum Associated, Sussex

Newton C (1991) *The Roper, Logan and Tierney Model in Action*. Macmillan, Basingstoke

Oijen E, Charnock A (1995) What is sexuality? *Nurs Times* **91**(17): 26–7

Piaget J (1951) cited in Rutter M (1971) Normal psychosexual development. *J Child Psychol Psychiatry* **11**: 259–83

Pletsch P, Johnson M, Tosi C, Thurston C, Riesch S (1991) Self-image among early adolescents: revisited. *J Comm Health Nurs* **8**(4): 215–31

Proctor M, Swinford T (1996) Expressing sexuality: Married with two children. *Assignment* **2**(2): 25–30

Rafferty D (1995) Putting sexuality on the agenda. *Nurs Times* **91**(17): 28–31

Roper N, Logan W, Tierney A (1980) *The Elements of Nursing*. Churchill Livingstone, Edinburgh

Rutter M (1971) Normal psychosexual development. *J Child Psychol Psychiatry* **11**: 259–83

Stainland J, Newell R (1996) Adolescent attitudes to sex education. *Br J Sex Med* **23**: 12–18

Webb C (1985) *Sexuality, Nursing and Health*. John Wiley and Sons, Chichester

Welling K, Wadsworth J, Johnson A, Field J, Whitaker L, Field B (1995) Provision of sex education and early sexual experience: The relation examined. *Br Med J* 311: 417–20

7
The pregnant adolescent: sexually ignorant or destroyer of societies values?

Tessa Muncey

'Trusting his images, he assumes their relevance,
Mistrusting my images, I question their relevance.

Assuming their relevance, he assumes the fact,
Questioning their relevance, I question the fact'.

(Robert Graves, 1986)

Graves' poem 'Broken Images' provides the theme for a consideration of the reasons for adolescent pregnancy. The patriarchal child-rearing expert has portrayed an image of childhood that assumes relevance to everyone and provides a powerful catalogue of facts on which successful child-rearing should be based, mother-blaming being the ultimate sanction when things go wrong. As a feminist I mistrust the images and question the facts and their relevance given the hegemonic power[1] they endorse.

This chapter will consider the argument that early unplanned pregnancy is not just a matter of failed contraception or lack of sex education advice, but is part of the wider debate on childhood sexuality. Views that are aided and abetted by the myth of childhood happiness and endorsed by the child-rearing expert. The following case study will serve to illustrate my discomfort at some of the well-documented explanations that are put forward to explain it.

1. The health carers perspective

On April 22nd, a young woman was told that her pregnancy test was positive. She underwent a completely uneventful pregnancy which culminated in the birth of a very healthy baby boy on December 14th.

The girl was 15 years old. The midwife condemned her as a 'promiscuous young woman who failed to use contraceptives'. The social worker appointed to advise her said just give him up for adoption and get on with your life.

The father of the child was arrested but not charged with unlawful sexual intercourse.

---

1   Hegemony describes the complex processes through which a ruling class secures and maintains power over other social classes. It refers to the interrelationship of economic, political and social forces, the techniques of coercion and consent which guarantee the existing relations of production. For 'hegemony' to be secured everyone must accept, at the level of 'common-sense' knowledge, the view of the dominant class (Barrett, 1980).

2. The grandmother's tale

In an informal autobiography twenty-three years after this event, the girl's mother presented her with 'The Grandmother's Tale'. In it she had used her many talents to pass on fragments of her life. Photography, pressed flowers and calligraphy adorned a text that conjured up happy days amid the pleasures of the countryside. Wild flowers, walks, cycling all unfolding with a rosy glow of retrospection. Even the war set against the backdrop of the delights of new countryside when evacuated to a first teaching post in Worcestershire. However, she reports that:

> "The twelve years of country plenty were followed by ten leaner one's back in town — out of our natural element perhaps so many things seem to go wrong' ... but it was not to be forever. We decided to move and looked around for a new country cottage'.

3. The girl's story

In those ten lean years, the girl was subjected to repeated incestuous sexual abuse. Her confusion increased, her self-esteem plummeted and she felt unable to tell anybody. Nobody seemed surprised when after a very successful junior school education she started to fail at school.

Sex became the currency of affection and nurturing and she glided effortlessly from sex at home to sex with others. Nobody asked the right questions that might have elicited the real problems. School blamed her for failing there. Family were content to let the early pregnancy be blamed as adolescent ignorance. What none of them saw was the bleak and twisted world of a girl whose self-esteem was so blighted by her experiences that the idea of a baby to care for was, in a naive way, a treat to look forward to. A girl for whom sexual practice had been a reality for years. An unspeakable kind of incestuous relationship about which there is no one to confide in.

This case study illustrates that all the actors in the drama of a teenage pregnancy have a perspective. In order to understand the nature of this 'tragedy', the discourse must take account of all the evidence. The typical assumptions of the first two perspectives are: that young people are supposed to be asexual and innocent and childhood is filled with happy, non-sexual activities until a life partner has been selected, at an age that society deems to be mature and financially responsible. If pregnancy occurs before this time, then it is clearly ignorance or the girl herself has just made a silly mistake. The girl's own story demonstrates the hidden characteristics of this, otherwise, quite straightforward history.

Adolescent pregnancy: just a failure of contraception?

Pregnancy is seen as an aberration in society's expected pattern of adolescent behaviour. Theoretical explanations that are put forward to explain it tend not to reflect the whole range of features depicted in the case study. The discourse on adolescent pregnancy is polarised between several factions, each claiming to have the causes of early pregnancy clearly established and campaigning vociferously for support for their solutions. However, it will become apparent that most of them find the young girl herself culpable, and none really considers that there may be a more obvious underlying problem. The most popular ideas that will be explored are:

1. The young pregnant adolescent is not only held responsible for the moral decline in society, particularly the threat to the nuclear family, but deliberately acts to obtain welfare benefits by deception.
2. Sex education paradoxically encourages sexuality in the innocent, happy child and yet lack of it increases the likelihood of pregnancy.
3. Adolescent pregnancy carries considerable health risks and causes educational failure and poverty.

The underlying assumptions about the nature of childhood are very pervasive. It is purported that children are innocent, happy and asexual. The more insidious links between childhood sexual victimisation and early pregnancy are so contrary to this view that they rarely occur in the same discourse.

An exploration of the myth of childhood happiness will follow an overview of the discrepancies and inadequacies of the prominent arguments, and lead on to a consideration of childhood sexual victimisation. The contribution of the child-rearing expert and a stylised imagery of childhood to the idealised viewpoint will lead, inexorably, to the conclusion that understanding the nature of childhood sexuality must begin by asking different questions. Instead of asking, 'Why do young girls get pregnant' it might be more pertinent to ask, 'Why do young girls engage in sexual activity?' Even the advocates of early sex education take it as read that young girls are engaging in early sexual activity and, rather than investigate the reasons for this, they argue strongly for increased sex education at an early age. (Marot, 1994).

In the 1990s, girls start their menstrual cycles as early as nine years old (Cook, 1995). This has led to a lowering of the age at which young girls become pregnant, illustrated by the nine-year-old who gave birth in 1996. Can this really be explained as 'a biological urge for sexual gratification at puberty, which is so strong that the risk of parenthood is often forgotten in the excitement (Ranjan, 1993), or Sayer's suggestion that 'most of the teenagers who engage in sexual activity are in it for the same reasons as most adults: for the loving arms, the warmth, the reassurance that one matters, and the comfort, the touching and the skin to skin communication just like an adult'? (Sayer, 1982).

Health risks

Inherent in these arguments is the view that adolescent pregnancy is a problem for society in general, for the health of the young girl in particular and inevitably leads to legal wrangles, involving protracted debates about the age of consent and the medical professions responsibilities in administering contraceptives.

Each problem is considered in isolation, doctors and midwives emphasising the health risks from early pregnancy. Obstetricians focus on the maternal, fetal and neonatal risks that are highest at the extremes of the reproductive age. Conception under the age of 16 years is associated with an increased perinatal death rate and with an increase in the rate of premature deliveries (Royal College of Obstetricians and Gynaecologists, 1991). Ranjan (1993) even goes so far as to suggest that 'the impact of pregnancy at such a tender age far outweighs any ethical, moral or legal consideration'. Such is the concern of doctors for young girls' health that the Department of Health (1992) has identified teenage pregnancy as one of the aspects of health, which needs to be tackled on an urgent basis in the Government's White Paper, *The Health of the Nation*. In England and Wales in 1993, 8.1 in every 1000 young women aged 13–15 years became pregnant. In Scotland, the figure is slightly less at 8 in every 1000 (Brooks Advisory Centre, 1996). Approximately half of the pregnancies among under 16-year-olds ends in abortion. The Health of the Nation set a target to halve the pregnancy rate in this age group by the year 2000 from 9.5 per 1000 13–15-year-olds in 1989 to no more than 4.8 (Department of Health, 1992). What these figures do not reveal is the number of young girls engaging in sexual intercourse who do not get pregnant or those that miscarry.

This view is fraught with contradictions. Despite the argument that teenage pregnancy is likely to have a higher mortality and morbidity rate, this is explainable in that pregnant teenagers are late bookers and poor attenders in antenatal care, often concealing their pregnancy to the detriment of their own and their baby's health by missing out on vital antenatal screening. They may smoke, consume alcohol, take inappropriate medication and have poor nutritional understanding. Makinson (1985) suggests that the consequences of teenage pregnancy and childbirth and the increased risk of maternal complications is largely related to social and economic origins. Problems associated with such health risks include: low socio-economic status, unemployment, welfare dependency, bad housing and social environment, isolation and depression, low educational achievement and lack of support from a stable relationship. Problems that are not unlike those caused by pregnancy at any age in women with similar histories. As already stated, it is girls with these types of problems who appear statistically more likely to progress with their pregnancies. It is more likely that girls from the higher socio-economic groups will be pressed into abortions and may suffer physiological and psychological problems as a result, but who are not deemed a drain on society's scarce resources in order to support the child. If the welfare system then imposes further restrictions by limiting benefits, it is actually exacerbating the problem not alleviating it. After all in 1994 there were 7200 pregnancies in the under-16-year-olds and more than half of these ended in abortion (Hadley, cited in Cassidy, 1995). This does not represent a significant drain on the benefits bill. What it does do, in line with the Criminal Justice Act, is put the problem back onto the shoulders of the parents. The mortality and morbidity rates of adolescent pregnancies could fall dramatically if the stigma and financial burden were removed from young people. As a health visitor, I witnessed the Catch 22 situation of young mothers who were denied access to housing on the grounds that they were not eligible until they had a live birth, who were then given the added burden of trying to learn how to run a home, establish a relationship with their child and eke out a living on the pittance offered to them by the state, all at the same time. A false economy when the long-lasting health consequences of poverty far outweigh any cost that could have been used in preventative action.

Moral decline

While the medical fraternity deliberates over the health of the young girl and her baby, the politicians express concern over the demise of family life and its effects on the moral decay within society. Single parenthood is the focus of British government interest for four main reasons: the implications for social security spending; concerns for the welfare of their children; fears that these children will go on to be delinquent; and fears that a 'cycle of deprivation' will lead to the creation of an 'underclass' which threatens society (Doherty, 1995). Politicians, such as Michael Howard, have moralised that 'so called 'progressive' theories in the sixties and seventies made excuses for crime . . . some parents neglected the difference between right and wrong'. (Howard, *Independent on Sunday*, 1993). Part of this story has been the decline in the traditional two-parent family. More recently, John Redwood has suggested that the babies born to young mothers should be placed for adoption not just because the numbers available have decreased over the years but to reduce benefit handouts (Cassidy, 1995). However, the common stereotype of young women becoming pregnant in order to obtain welfare benefits and housing has been shown to be unfounded as births to young women living in poverty do not decline or increase with changes in welfare policies and payments (Anon, *Daily Telegraph*, 1982; Furstenberg *et al*, 1981; Clark, 1989; Phoenix, 1993).

Political action translates itself into law, and a picture emerges of what is perceived as normal. The British government's ideal of family life is that a mature man and woman meet, they fall in love, they get married, they have children, the man provides for the family by working and the woman stays at home to care for the children. These ideals are not necessarily consistent with reality and Hutter and Williams (1981) suggest they demonstrate the covert forms of control exerted on all women. From this Doherty suggests a set of contradictory expectations arise.

- thou shalt not get pregnant — thou shalt not use contraception: child bearing outside marriage is wrong, but to have sex outside marriage, women must be swept away by love. Only 'slags' carry and use contraception
- thou shalt have children — thou shalt not keep an illegitimate baby: a women's biological destiny is motherhood, but a single woman who becomes pregnant must have an abortion or offer the child for adoption
- thou shalt not be socially dependent — thou shalt stay at home with the children: it is wrong to depend on state benefits for a living, but the 'good mother' does not abandon her children to go out to work
- thou shalt be rational — thou shalt be irrational: women must be rational in deciding not to become single mothers, but are slaves to their passions in love, and to their hormones in wanting children. They cannot legally decide to have an abortion and, to be granted one, a doctor must typically assess them as psychologically unstable.

Sexually ignorant

Further to this view of the pernicious single parent is another common stereotype put forward by politicians — that of the young women who is ignorant or indifferent to contraceptive use. The aim of the *Health of the Nation* to reduce teenage pregnancies contains the uncontested assumption that behaviour is based on rationality. This is rather the 'logical rationalisation' of the average white male politician (Doherty, 1995). Doherty goes on to outline some of the other elements in a woman's decision-making process. The perceived costs and benefits of contraceptive use; costs and benefits of pregnancy; the likelihood of pregnancy; and the availability of facilities for pregnancy terminations (Luker, 1975; 1977; cited in Doherty, 1995). Unprotected intercourse may occur because of the cost of contraception or the difficulty in obtaining it or even the stigmatisation of carrying condoms and the embarrassment of negotiating their use (Boyle, 1991). Teenagers also underestimate their own chances of conceiving (Morrison, 1985; Littlejohn, 1992; Cvetkovich and Grote, 1981). The romantic imagery of motherhood as the ultimate fulfilment may actually override Luker's pragmatic rationality (Prendergast and Prout, 1980; Oakley, 1981).

Wendy Hollway (1989) also challenges 'the dominant western assumption of the rational unitary subject' when she suggests, in a framework of structural linguistics, that making love without contraception can come to signify 'securing commitment to a relationship'. Young women's decisions then can be seen to be shaped by practical considerations, emotions and social pressures.

While the government sees pregnancy in young girls leading to limiting educational experience and a drain on limited government resources, the evidence would suggest that young girls who get pregnant are already failing at school, come from backgrounds where their self-esteem is not developed at home and they are looking for alternatives (Crouch, cited by Cassidy, 1995). Mills found in her study of teenage attitudes to pregnancy in Glasgow that 'sexual activity was one way to pass the time if unemployed' (Mills, 1988). In this particular area of high unemployment, poor housing, and with high rates of drug abuse and crime, having a baby was one way of giving and receiving love if they came from an unloving home. In a life with very few choices, sex was something that girls could say yes to and enjoy with very little initial outlay. In the *Bristol Booking Survey* in 1980, fewer than one in six teenage mothers had 'O' levels and nearly one third were without any measurable educational attainment. These girls were also likely to come from broken homes and be low achievers. There appears to be a strong correlation between low income and high rates of contraceptive failure (Family Planning Association, 1980).

The paradox of sex education and legal prohibitions

Despite the apparent concern by the government to reduce teenage pregnancies and the evidence that suggests that improved sex education decreases teenage pregnancy rates, why is sex education in the school curriculum only a recommendation? The importance of education is as preparation for adult life but not in this important field. On the one hand there are people who suggest that encouraging sexual awareness at an early age invites experimentation and, on the other, there are the parents, who for a variety of reasons, believe these issues should remain in the control of parents. This despite the fact that in the Netherlands, where contraception and sex education are more readily available, teenage pregnancy rates are much lower (Scally, 1992). Many parents have inhibitions about sex or do not have adequate experience of how to approach the subject easily. They may leave explanations until too late, when the adolescent is less responsive to parental influence (Cook, 1995).

Society tries to discourage adolescent pregnancies by ineffective legal prohibitions which clearly do not deter them; more than ever girls as young as 12 years admit to being sexually active whether by consent or compliance. Sexuality of young people leads to ambiguities. In 1994 the headlines of some newspapers screamed outrage at the proposed publication of a guide to safer sex for 16–24-year-olds by the Health Education Authority. The 'Your Pocket Sex Guide' was withdrawn. Journalists also revealed that health promotion workers were handing out free condoms to under 16s as part of a health initiative. This moral outrage ignores the fact that it is not illegal to provide any form of contraception to under 16s. Where there has always been confusion, ambiguity and inhibition in discussions about contraception and sex for young people, the situation was made more difficult by the confusion surrounding the Gillick case. Youth policy is often constructed to meet the needs of adults. The law sets the age of consent to sexual intercourse at 16 years. In 1969 The Family Law Reform Act set the age of medical majority at 16 years. In 1980 the Department of Health and Social Security set out the following principles; that young people should have the right to confidentiality, the right to decide to inform their parents and, if under the age of 16 years, general practitioners could decide whether or not to inform parents. Victoria Gillick, a mother of 10 from Norfolk, challenged her health authority on the grounds that it deprived her of her parental rights. Although the subsequent ruling in 1985 by the Law Lords overturned her appeal, they pronounced by a majority of 3:2 that 'Gillick competence' must be proved in order to justify overriding the wishes of parents. Gillick competence is stated '. . . as a matter of law the parental right to determine whether or not their minor child below the age of 16 will have medical treatment terminates if and when the child achieves a sufficient understanding and intelligence to enable him or her to understand fully what is proposed . . . until the child achieves the capacity to consent, the parental right continues. (Gillick, 1986). (Interestingly, the same competence does not apply to withdrawal from treatment as in the case of the young girl who wanted to refuse treatment for her anorexia.) This has led to uncertainty about their rights and GPs are now more likely to be cautious as a result. Probably less well known are the Fraser Guidelines that were issued by Lord Fraser following the House of Lords ruling in the case of Gillick. The Fraser Guidelines suggest that a doctor may give contraceptive advice or treatment to young people under 16 years of age, if the doctor is satisfied that all the following requirements are fulfilled:

- the young person understands the doctor's advice
- the doctor cannot persuade the young person to inform his or her parents or allow the doctor to inform the parents that he or she is seeking contraceptive advice
- the young person is very likely to begin or continue having intercourse with or without contraceptive treatment
- unless he or she receives contraceptive advice or treatment, the young person's physical or mental health or both are likely to suffer
- the young person's best interests require the doctor to give contraceptive advice, treatment or both without parental consent.

More simply in Scotland, the Medical Defence Union has advised that doctors may give contraceptive advice or treatment to young people under 16 years of age, without their parents knowing, if they cannot persuade the young person to inform his or her family.

As a result of the uncertainty that the Gillick ruling brought, a consumer test carried out by the Brook Advisory Centre, published in a report in 1992, showed that 44% of teenagers requesting help from family planning clinics found negative attitudes. The rise in the teenage birth-rate in the 1980s, following a noticeable fall in the previous decade, can be attributed somewhat to the effects of this confusion as well as to economic recession and family planning cuts (Cassidy, 1995).

The legislative focus serves to reinforce the stereotypes of promiscuity and permissiveness that are associated with adolescent sexuality. However, sexuality is not the only example of status ambiguity. Two recent acts that are diametrically opposed to each other, The Children Act 1989 and The Criminal Justice Act 1991 indicate the ambiguities in relation to young people and the law. The Children Act proposes that: Children and young people should have a voice of their own, be treated as individuals with rights and responsibilities. eg. if boys or girls have the maturity to understand the implications of their decision they can change their name, religion etc. On the other hand, the Criminal Justice Act proposes that the behaviour of children is the responsibility of their parents. How to determine maturity is the greatest limitation of these acts and they sit uneasily with other ambiguities in civil status: At 17 years of age an adolescent can join the army and be killed fighting, drive most vehicles, buy a fire arm and hold a pilot's licence yet cannot vote, serve on a jury or make a will and at 16 years of age they can marry, join a trade union and live in a brothel, but they cannot be tattooed, own a house or a flat or use a porn shop.

The Criminal Justice Act 1991 strengthens already existing legislation by:

a) requiring a parent or guardian to attend court with a young person;

b) creating powers to make a parent or guardian responsible for financial penalties imposed by the court; and

c) enabling the court to bind over the parent or guardian as a result of offences committed by the young person. In short designed to ensure delay in development, young people are the property and responsibility of parents.

The law then seeks to maintain hegemonic control, by reinforcing control of certain behaviours by certain groups of people. The law is not enabling, it seeks to set moral standards that are outside its remit with an over-reliance on adult informants and adult-based paradigms.

Social control of this kind is non-rational and leads to policy contradictions, such as the attempts to limit contraceptive advice to under 16-year-olds and making sex education discretionary, while trying to reduce teenage pregnancies. The major source of inconsistency is the attempt to deny women's sexuality, the idea that sex has to be legitimised only as procreation, which is legitimised by marriage, which is legitimised by love. (Doherty, 1995). However, it is difficult to reconcile the legislation with adolescents in general when most of the problems relate to young women in particular. Is the government purposely trying to suppress or control the sexuality of women? It is hard not to arrive at this conclusion when boys' responsibility for pregnancy has declined since the advent of the contraceptive pill. One unique ruling in the Appeal Court in 1989 overruled a 17-year-old boy's attempt to gain custody of his own child (Kirby, 1989). The court concluded that the baby would be better off adopted than with his natural father. This ruling presumably occurred because the natural mother wanted to give the child up for adoption, although it is open to doubt whether she would have been forbidden by law to raise her own child, whatever her age, on the grounds that she may lose interest as it was deemed the father might. There is very little research about teenage fathers, although the statistical evidence suggests that teenage marriages are vulnerable and experts generally agree that boys mature more slowly than girls. The underlying assumption is that girls generally have some kind of innate, instinctive, nurturing qualities, allowing them to be mothers at any age, but boys do not. The need to justify a boy's desire to raise his child is mirrored in the strenuous regulations that adoptive parents have to undergo in order to prove their worthiness to become parents, as opposed to the total absence of any rules for natural parents to do the same.

Adolescent pregnancy is often viewed as a problem for society. It is considered an indication of a society that is spiralling out of control in the wake of the decline of the nuclear family. Much of the rationale for prevention is thinly disguised as concern for the health of the young girl and her baby, wrapped up in arguments about the legal status of the child or rights and responsibilities of parents. The sum total of these debates is confusion and a lack of clarity in the professions' responsibilities in administering contraceptives and health advice. What rarely happens in the debate is for all the issues to be considered in a wider context, or for the rhetoric to be discarded in favour of the voices of the young people themselves.

The picture emerges of a group of young women who are heavily targeted as a problem, for whom the solutions contain many contradictions. These contradictions seem destined to make the situation worse by acting more as a punishment than a deterrent, and they avoid addressing relevant issues rather than enlightening the women through education.

What appears to be missing from the debate is a sense of the reality from the young person's perspective. There seems to be a serious attempt to deny the sexuality of young people and cloak their lives in a rhetoric that endorses the myth of childhood happiness. There is an assumption that sex and pregnancy are inextricably linked in the minds of young girls, whereas many suggest they felt pressurised into 'having sex' by their peers and by moral blackmail from their boyfriends who threatened to leave them if they did not comply (Mills, 1988). A power struggle develops and pregnancy is the by-product, signalling an unhealthy attitude to sexuality, which results from low self-esteem rather than a conscious decision to get pregnant. This is incompatible with health education about contraception or laws that suggest that underage sex is illegal.

Early forced sexual intercourse

In questioning some of the assumptions about sexual behaviour in general and pregnancy in particular, the evidence that is less well publicised is the relationship between childhood sexual abuse and early sexual activity. A number of studies demonstrate the disproportionately large numbers of young women who become pregnant during adolescence, and who report that they were the victims of childhood sexual abuse. (Gershenson *et al*, 1989; Butler and Burton, 1990; Boyer and Fine, 1992; Stevens-Simon and Reichert, 1994). These figures are usually under reported as a result of many difficulties, not least of which is that girls fear they will not be believed. So the 50–60% of girls who become pregnant and who do report sexual abuse may not be a true representation.

Epidemiological studies suggest that between 15% and 38% of women in the general population have had unwanted sexual contact before 18 years of age (Bachman *et al*, 1988; Finkelhor, 1986; Russell, 1983; Wyatt, 1985). Estimates for childhood sexual abuse are set as high as 1:3 for girls and 1:7 for boys (Bass and Davis, 1988).

The impact of this early abuse has a measurable effect on psychological functioning, behavioural choices and social adjustment (Lanz, 1995). It could, therefore, be argued that pregnancy is just a manifestation of self-destructive and socially-deviant patterns of behaviour associated with sexual victimisation, rather than the origin of these behaviours (Rainey *et al*, 1995).

In America, links are currently being made between prostitution and pornography, and the victims of incest, but attempts to do so in Britain are being strenuously denied or played down (Dellacoste and Alexander, 1987). Could it be that the real solution in preventing childhood pregnancies is to face the greatest taboo of all — incest. It could be that the only reason pregnancy does not occur before the age of nine is that it is not yet possible. The onset of puberty has dramatically increased over the last few years as a direct result of increased nutrition. The implication is that as the age of puberty has decreased so the 'biological urge for sexual gratification, which can be so strong that the risk of parenthood is often forgotten in the heat of the moment' (Ranjan, 1993), has also decreased. Is it a serious proposition that this statement really applies to a nine-year-old girl? What seems more likely is that the girl has been subjected to sexual behaviour from an early age, which for her has become the norm, and then she finds it difficult to distinguish between normal loving, trusting childhood friendships and sex and betrayal. Needs for nurturing become confused with sex. An interesting feature of child abuse cases that never come to court, is that the long-term effects that can afflict a survivor are often the very attributes of the 'bad witness' which cause the cases to be thrown out by the Department of Public Prosecutions: attributes, such as promiscuity, prostitution and substance abuse.

Deeply held assumptions about childhood sexuality have been incorporated into the collective unconscious by the steady and insistent flow of knowledge conveyed by the child-rearing experts. Gradually, the whole moral, legal and economic climate of our society has become imbued by the patriarchal authority of the, mainly male, psychologist.

Child-rearing experts and the myth of childhood happiness

> '*Childhood is only the beautiful and happy time in contemplation and retrospect: to the child it is full of deep sorrows, the meaning of which is unknown*'.
>
> (George Eliot, cited in Paterson, 1928)

> '*Adults have implicit theories about what children are like, about the causes of children's behaviour and about the way which children should be trained*'.
>
> (Wegner and Vallacher, 1977)

The separate sphere of childhood has grown — as a social concept, as a market possibility, as an area of research, as a problem. Children are no longer chattels and new legal measures, such as the Children's Act, give them voice in choices and decision-making about their legal situation (Warner, 1994). What is looked for in children may be determined by what you expect to find; and what you expect to find is very much determined by the insistent ebb and flow of nineteenth and twentieth century discourses about childhood and its relationship to adulthood.

Child-rearing is often considered to be 'common-sense'. Parenting skills are not taught in the way that other subjects are in schools, with many parents taking a 'trial-and-error' approach to child-rearing. These approaches are a culmination of ideas, based on memories of their own childhood upbringing with: advice from families, first hand experience of children, direct influence of members of household, eg. grandparents, family folklore, traditions of the community, personal contact with, and observation of, other people and their ideas, information and advice as presented in books and other media, 'second hand' experiences, films, plays, books, magazines, religious or spiritual teachings and evidence from research. Although last in a long list, the influence of research on the implicit psychology of most people is perhaps the most important. So, too, is the unspoken triadic relationship between theory, particularly psychological theory, social policy and practice, and political priorities.

Our assumptions about the capacities of children affect what we expect of them and what we offer them. Our beliefs about children's needs give us the assurance that we know what to expect and how to rear them. But there is need for caution, as these images and beliefs are ways of rationalising practices, the origins of which go back into history and culture.

The centrality of the child-rearing expert in family life is essentially a nineteenth century phenomenon. De Mause (1974) asserts that, historically, child-rearing was a catalogue of atrocities, including infanticide to dispose of unwanted children, and there seems to be no doubt that children were often neglected and exploited in the past. In a critique of four significant studies of childhood, Stone (1981) concludes that it is difficult to study children in isolation without considering how parents treated children. The critical change to more affectionate parent-child relationships seems to have taken place in the eighteenth century.

Whatever the historical viewpoint, there is no doubt that the twentieth century has become the century of the child in Britain. At the turn of the eighteenth century, children did not command much attention; women had, on average, seven births and a third or a half would not live beyond the age of five years. By 1900 infant mortality was declining due to improvements in nutrition and sanitation. Birthrates dropped to an average of 3.5, children were expected to live and contraception became more available. Economic changes also pushed the child into prominence when production left the household, thus sweeping away many of the chores that had filled the child's day, and childhood began to figure as a distinct and fascinating phase of life. Child labour had its ideological defenders, educational philosophers who extolled the lessons of factory discipline, and others who argued that a father had a patriarchal right to dispose of his child's labour. However, the reform-oriented middle classes were horrified by the hunched and rickety children, blinded by fine work and lungs ruined by coal dust. So part of the focus on childhood became an assertion of what were thought to be traditional human values against the horrors of capitalism. But, more than this, the child became the symbol of the industrial future. The child became the reason to seek reforms. Due to its ability to learn and pliancy, the child would be the only member of the family who could be prepared for the technological turmoil of the outside world.

Mother as guardian of the race

This ideology raised the status of motherhood to a higher level. As the person who was biologically responsible for producing the child, the mother was held responsible for its development. Ellen Key (1909), in her best seller 'The Century of the Child', suggested that women would have more effect in transforming the world through child-rearing than entering parliament or journalism. This was at a time when women were campaigning for the vote. Motherhood was established as an important role. In 1894, a women's magazine implores the mother to reconcile her own inherited precepts with modern ideas and grasp firmly the idea that 'At all costs her children must learn obedience, for obedience is the very religion of childhood, and is the beginning of all the morality and self-restraint, which are so hardly learnt later, when the pampered will is weak from want of training', (Anon, 1894). Inherent in this assertion are all the Victorian ideologies of sexuality which had been created by the moral panics of the time. The fears generated by the French Revolution significantly shaped Victorian sexuality. English politicians feared that socialism would spread like a malignancy from France where the sexual excesses of prostitutes were regarded as the vanguard of socialism. Blaming the victim, sexual deviancy, sexually-transmitted diseases and unemployment were the signs of a society spiralling out of control and the woman was to maintain her rightful place as 'Angel in the House' to bolster the failing moral standards. Mothers had to be wise, unselfish and brave and many seemed to be proud of such a respected position. Motherhood was not a part-time job or a biological condition but a noble calling. This official ideology, powerfully controlled by legislation and social practices embodied in the concept of marriage, condemned the woman and her children to the 'private sphere', and separated them from the man's 'public sphere' of work. Within this 'private sphere' the child is left, but because of the importance of the child as a prototype for the society of the future, man realises that she should not be left alone. The rapid rise of the child-rearing expert reflected the growing prestige of experts in other areas of women's lives. The male take-over of healing had created a model for professional authority in all areas of domestic activity. The experts did not come uninvited, some young mothers near the turn of the century refused to see child-rearing as instinctive and were eager to defer to the experts trained in child study. With the separation of private and public realms, the standards of 'success' in child-raising came to be set outside the home beyond the mother's control. Child-rearing had always had a class emphasis, the working classes needing to provide a future work force with relevant skills and the discipline to keep home industries going, or to provide workers to support the aristocracy. Industrialisation, however, increased the proportion of people in the middle-classes who were more concerned with equipping young women with housewifery skills and encouraging young men to follow in their father's footsteps. Paradoxically the 'better' the mother, the more home-oriented she is, the less experience she will have in the outside world where her efforts will be judged. It was a question of great concern as to how women could raise boys to be men. It is this notion of difference between the genders and the different needs in the child-rearing process that are central to the 'Oedipal Complex' at the heart of Freud's psycho-dynamic model (Freud, 1940). The model depends on a particular, gendered organisation in the division of labour in society and yet the continuance of a belief in the differences between the genders depends on Freud's ideas. The mother is required to create a sexual division of psychic organisation and orientation that produces men and women who enter into asymmetrical heterosexual relationships. It produces men who react to fear and act superior to women (Chodorow, 1978). This placed a great deal of responsibility on the mother and at her feet could be placed the blame if the final outcome was flawed.

Scientific motherhood

Women gathered to discuss and confront the problems posed by their new situation, but did not seem to challenge the situation itself. The National Congress of Mothers in 1897 concerned itself with the preservation of the home and were concerned by the 'tide of femininity' which was streaming towards a career. The concern was that mothering was not enough for some women. One immediate solution seemed to be to reinterpret motherhood as a profession requiring degrees and licences and open only to those who could demonstrate fitness. The birth of the professional mother was overshadowed by the child-rearing expert from the discipline of psychology. This discipline was applying the paradigm of science. Scientific motherhood included the laws of human development and nutrition. The goal was industrial man and, in the interests of industrial regularity, spontaneity would have to be subdued, good habits and regularity must be established, starting with physical habits, such as eating sleeping and bowel movements. The hygienist movement started by Truby King (Mander, 1996), a New Zealand psychologist, is epitomised by an entry in *Maternity and Child Welfare*, a monthly journal for workers among mothers and children. 'Habits are the result of repeated action. The baby is born without habits, and what habits he may develop, whether they are good or bad habits, depends usually on the mother or those who are responsible for his care' (Allen de Villbiss, 1920), essential habits being focused on regular feeding, personal cleanliness and regular bowels, active exercise, prompt obedience and plenty of fresh air. These ideas mirrored the increasing interest in Behaviourism, which set out to refute mind-soul subjectivity and consciousness. Philosophical ideas, traditionally attributed to John Locke, suggested that babies are born, not with a strong will in the traditional Christian view reinforced by Calvinist theology of the notion of 'original sin', but in a state 'void of all character' or with a 'tabula rasa' (Russell, 1946). Nothing disturbed Watson (1928) more than the irrational, emotional elements in the mother-child relationship, in particular the issue of women raising men, but while Watson was accepting the limitations of the middle-class home, a more serious menace lurked in the neighbourhoods of the poor. Child-rearing was set to extend itself as a tool for potential social control. Expertise had to be disseminated more widely if the lower social classes with their irrational child-rearing methods were not to threaten the fabric of industrial life.

Although Watson's ideas achieved a prominence in the scientific world that psychology was trying to break into, it was Freud's ideas that continued to have a very powerful effect on attitudes to children and sexuality in particular.

Childhood sexuality

Freud wrote about some psychical consequences of the anatomical distinctions between the sexes. His investigations were not really centred on the gender role or gender identity as was the Behaviourist movement, but how these two anatomically distinct groups develop different kinds of mental lives and have different experiences. He did not question that these behavioural and psychical differences existed. Central to Freud's ideas of gender difference is the Oedipus Complex. Children with penises undergo a different type of fantasy experience, which culminates in incorporating the values and behaviours appropriate to his gender through fear of rejection and castration. Girls, on the other hand, when they realise that they are different from their fathers, start to identify with their mothers. The psychologising of physical attributes was a central tenet of Freud's ideas. He had worked alongside Dr Charcot, one of the first men to believe that women's hysteria was not a product of the wandering womb as had previously been thought, but that physical symptoms had psychological origins. In April 1896 Freud presented a paper to his colleagues at the Society for Psychiatry and Neurology in Vienna, in which he postulated the seduction theory, that the origins of hysteria lay in early sexual traumas, incestuous rape visited by fathers on daughters or even mothers on sons. He concluded that, contrary to the belief of the abusers themselves, sexual abuse in childhood had the most profound and lifelong traumatic effects on victims. Due to the cool reception that these ideas received, nine years later, in 1905, he publicly retracted the seduction theory arguing that he had been deceived. The first evidence of False Memory Syndrome was recorded when he recognised that these scenes of seduction had never taken place and that they were only fantasies which his patient had made up. In order to explain this change of heart, he interwove the morality of the time concerning incest and masturbation into the belief that adults repressed memories of these activities and 'reworked' them into the unconscious, ascribing their sexual feelings at such a young age to childhood rape. It would appear that if Freud had not abandoned his seduction theory, his most significant contribution to twentieth-century thought would not have developed. Ideas such as the Oedipus and Electra complexes, that children from their earliest infancy are sexual beings, that repression can occur or even that the unconscious exists at all. The change of direction was incorporated into the psychological establishment and produced a powerful model for childhood sexuality until 1970 when Shulamith Firestone (1979) posited the idea that the armies of young women analysed by Freud and his followers may have been telling the truth and had actually, not metaphorically, been raped by their fathers. In her subsequent rejection of psychoanalysis, Alice Miller (1992) went further and suggested that Freud's real crime was to not be able to confront the truth about his own childhood. What was at first considered the expression of a personal flight from truth would be bought and sold all over the world as scientific truth. Alice Miller has recently dedicated herself to breaking down the wall of silence that she believes hides the 'scandalous, painful realities of childhood that therapies, such as psychoanalysis, have actually helped to contain and minimise. By seeking to explain everything in terms of repression, it is possible to consistently refuse to accept that parents are capable of routinely torturing their children. Therapists become trapped by the morality of the age they practice in and, instead of offering help to patients to resolve the consequences of the traumatisation that they have suffered, the therapists offer traditional morality, eg. forgiveness is presumed to be a condition for 'successful' therapy. Survivors of abuse are, therefore, encouraged not to blame others, but to take responsibility for their own healing by forgiveness.

Mother-blaming

Mother-blaming has emanated from psychoanalytic theories. A suspicion arose that women were not really natural mothers. Psychoanalysts peered into the rosy picture of the mother-child relationship and found a core of hideous pathology. Symptoms such as destructive, withdrawn, frightened, disturbed children emerged in place of the mutual bliss that mother and child were supposed to enjoy. Instead of blaming the isolation and solitude in which most women now had to raise their children, the experts agreed it must be the mother who was failing. If things did not improve despite copious advice to correct her faulty technique, then it must be faulty unconscious motivations. In the 1950s, Bowlby made devastating accusations against the rejecting mother. The mother who harboured hostile and rejecting feelings for her child was planting the seeds of neurosis, maternal deprivation and overprotectiveness, key features of 'bad mothers' (Bowlby, 1951). It took time for critics to recognise the juxtaposition of the socio-economic situation, the politics and psychological contributions that gave rise to these ideas. In the 1950s, just after the war, concern was expressed that women, who had entered the workplace to support the war effort, were not returning to their rightful place of work in the home to provide a haven for their families. Men returning from the war were finding it increasingly difficult to find work and what better way to get women back into the domestic sphere than by guilt. Mothering, for many years related to instincts via the work of ethnologists such as Lorenz, was now being raised as an important link in attachment. The maternally-deprived child could become at best over-demanding and unforgiving, but at worst an affectionless psychopath or juvenile delinquent. Thus began 40 years of policies that placed the needs of the child at the centre of decision-making in society, that treated them as innocent victims of adult behaviour and yet never really gave them any rights or took what they said seriously. Warner suggests that the injured child has become today's icon of humanity, an icon of which the phantom face of James Bulger has become the most haunting image of present horrors and social failure (Warner, 1994). However, many of these problems result from the concept that childhood and adult life are separate when they are in effect inextricably intertwined.

Parenting as an interactive process is perhaps best epitomised by the writings of Dr Spock (1979). He epitomised a move away from the rigidity of the industrial approach of behaviourism and rejected the intrinsically wilful child of psychodynamics. His was a child with a tendency towards goodness and healthy growth, underpinned by the philosophy of Rousseau (1762). Childhood was an important time when the behaviour of the child is appropriate to the needs and demands of the child's world and should be recognised and respected. Parents and teachers could distort and damage the natural progression towards goodness so must modify their activities to guide the natural development of the child. The child was an active agent in relation to the world rather than a passive recipient of experiences. Dr Spock's advice was that 'Your baby is born to be a reasonable, friendly human being' (Spock, 1946). Childcare focused on providing the right environment in which the child could explore and act out its predisposition to interact socially. The notion of the innocent, happy child is firmly entrenched in society's mind.

Childhood imagery

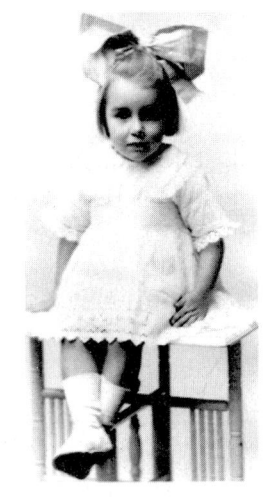

Nowhere is the myth of childhood innocence and happiness more established than in the family snapshot. One of the ways to understand childhood is to recall what it was like when we were young. Proust's (1984) literary evocation of childhood through adult memories is often quoted, but these involuntary memories have problems. They are selective, they may be fictional; how do we know they are 'from' not 'of' childhood?

Family snapshots are often used

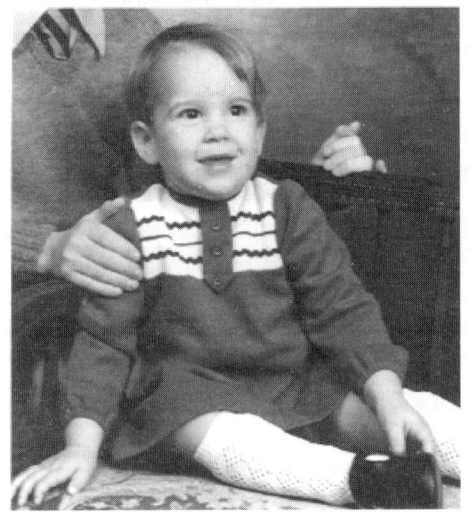

to evoke childhood memories, but interpreting them poses challenges. Our dreams of recalling a happy childhood and the need to belong, plus the selectivity of our memory causes fragmentation in the recollection of family histories. Yeats recalled in *Autobiographies*, his first memories were fragmentary and isolated as if time had not yet been created, all thoughts are connected with emotion and place without sequence. Family snapshots are

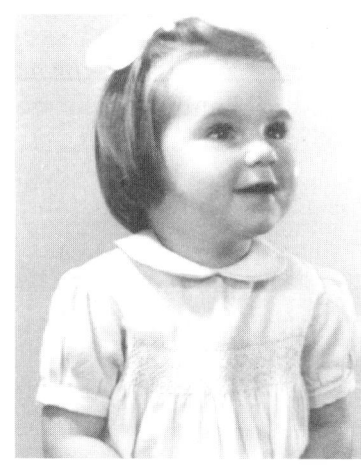

used to try and fill the gaps that memories leave out.

Spence and Holland (1991) refers to family photographs as symbolic images. The images of our families not only choose to immortalise each individual within a family but also betray the conventions of gender specific behaviours. Picture 1, 2 and 3 portrays images of three two-year-olds. They represent a very particular image of acceptable femininity despite a time span of 60 years between the photographs. All three are on some sort of pedestal, raised up as virtuous, innocent creatures that society has not yet defiled. Hair arranged and adorned by ribbons to add appeal. Pretty dresses, clean white socks, upward-turned smiling faces, the camera the same distance away, protecting their personal space, not too intrusive. Photography as a representation is referred to as the creation of a convincing illusion of reality. King (1992) suggests that photography is dominated by men and a masculine visual ideology creates an image to empower men as spectators, ie. they lay out things for them to desire. There is no evidence in any of these photos of the conflicts and anxieties, fears and desires that little girls may have. 'Family photography is an industry characterised by held off closure, happy beginnings, happy middles and no endings to all the family stories' (Kuhn, 1980).

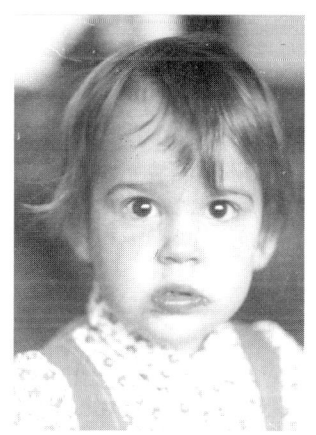

My memories of Rachel are recent and easy to recall. The still photograph does not capture her energy, characterised by constant movement and an insatiable desire for attention. Her brother's hand on her shoulder epitomises the grip of patriarchy as he exerts pressure in order to keep her still. She hardly ever wore a dress and white socks were soon dirtied. Picture 4 goes some way to explode this innocent, demure image by displaying a runny-nosed, dishevelled child who has clearly been crying and whose staring eyes straight to camera as opposed to averted, defies you not to take notice of her. The difference in style is attributed to the rationale for the photographs. The studio portraits are classic representations of little girls portraying an image that endorses society's expectations. Picture 4 on the other hand was taken by a photographer trying to subvert the stereotypical imagery.

The myth of childhood innocence

Feminists have tried to expose this myth of the innocent, non-sexual little girl. Sally Mann (1991) whose portraits of her children Emmett, Jessie and Virginia (see picture 5) take a very different view. Emmett is also two years old and her posture, head held back and hand on hip, characterises defiance. The photo is close up with her naked body displaying none of the trappings of stereotypical feminine adornment. In her pictures Mann attempts to demonstrate children growing up, their

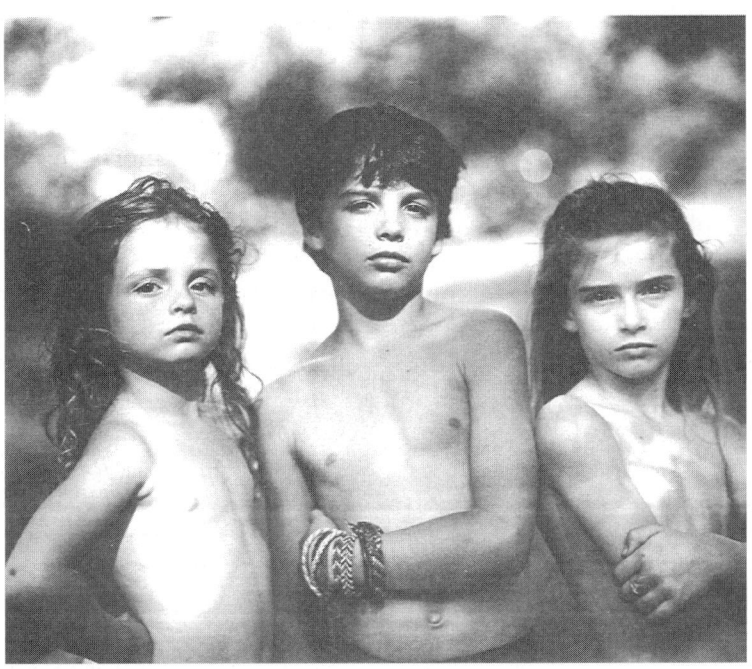

freedom and boldness constantly shadowed by dangers. She portrays hurt and damaged children, although she admits that the responsibility of judging nude or hurt children as art weighed against the conventional stance of parenting. Even here the ethos of 'bad mother' prevails. Bad mothers are those who let damage occur to the growing child; at best it should be avoided, at worst it should be concealed. There seems to be something morally permissible about portraying children of the destitute and starving in far off continents in the nude but not the well-fed offspring of the prosperous west. Sally Mann proves powerfully that family photos need not be naive chronicles of domestic idyll, but jealousy, anger and the inestimable danger of human relationships is played out in the arena of the home. 'In the risky intimacy of children and parents, adoration and terror are uneasy but inseparable companions' (Williams, 1992) In her response to this critique, Suzanne Moore (1992) suggests that these pictures expose the denial which society tries to maintain, that little girls are pre-sexual beings. Culturally we protect this image of innocence more effectively than we protect children, many of whom are abused in all sorts of ways.

Childhood depends for its meaning on its opposite to adulthood. Yet in reality these states are not so clearly demarcated. Just as adult models exploit the image of childhood to fantasise about powerlessness, children can portray precarious and seductive poses despite their lack of power. Exploitation of these images are the focus of pornographic imagery and is seen to flourish where there is a 'growing demand for fantasy fulfilment in the very heart of respectability' (Marcus, cited in Weeks, 1989). The principles of legal moralism [2] and legal paternalism [3] have been relied on by the conservatives to argue that good sex is always heterosexual, usually takes place within marriage and, if at all possible, is oriented towards procreation; and, more importantly sexually-explicit material activates 'all those polymorphous perverse snakes deep within us that threaten to undo civilisation in general and each of us in particular . . . and that the law ought to act as morality's handmaiden, protecting it from the forces of the flesh that would, if they could devour it.' (Tong, 1989). This very predictable debate has been shattered by a feminist contribution that seeks to expose pornography for what it is — the intentional degradation and subordination of women to men. As with the philosophical assumptions that underpin the advice from the child-rearing expert, the 'essentialist' view of sexuality as an overpowering force in the individual that shapes not only the personal but the social life as well, is a necessary assumption behind legal moralism and legal paternalism. Just as the prostitute became an object of fascination and disgust, ingrained in the public consciousness as a highly visible symbol of the social dislocation accompanying the new industrial era of the nineteenth century, paedophiles are contributing to questions about limits of sexual choice in the 1990s. The conceptualisation of the separateness of children appears to go hand in hand with the socially felt need to protect their

---

2   A person's liberty may be restricted to protect other specific individuals, but especially society as a whole from immoral behaviour where the word immoral means neither harmful or offensive but something like 'against a societal taboo' See Joel Feinberg (1973) *Social Philosophy* (Prentice-Hall, NJ) 36–41.

3   A person's liberty may be restricted to prevent him or herself from inflicted harm, or, in its extreme version, to guide that person, whether he or she likes it or not, towards his or her own good. See Joel Feinberg (1973) *Social Philosophy* (Prentice-Hall, NJ): 45–52.

purity and innocence. These ideas can be traced back to the greater emotional investment that accompanied the social construction of childhood in the nineteenth century. Ariès (1973) suggested in his work Centuries of Childhood, the idea of childhood did not exist in medieval society, there being no notion of intermediate stages between dependence and independence and the attainment of puberty was not signified by external manifestations of maturity. Weeks (1989) suggests that 'the separateness of childhood was axiomatic in Victorian ideology, a symbol of middle-class status as much as non-working women, and alongside this was an intensified emotional investment in the child and a fear of sexual corruption. Women were responsible for the purity of the home and private morality was the source and index of public morality. Freud discerned that the two erotic poles of Victorian men, idealisation and degradation were in fact complementary and that the romantic idealisation of the wife contributed to the necessity of prostitution (Corbin, 1990). It was in this greater emotional investment that Havelock Ellis (1936) and Freud (1977) were to 'discover' a childhood sexuality moulded within this intensified emotional harbour of the bourgeois family. However, Foucault suggests that sexual behaviour is organised through powers of incitement, definition and regulation. It is through ensembles of beliefs, concepts and organising ideas that our relation to reality is organised. This challenges the naturalness of what the middle-classes tried to convey as basic divisions (Foucault, 1977; cited in Weeks).

Woman as the tamer of men's sexuality

Havelock Ellis suggested that male sexuality was unproblematic, based as it was in the original primitive seizure of the female by the male. It was female sexuality that constituted the social problem because, through them, the race was perpetuated. (Havelock Ellis, 1936). So it is not just childhood sexuality that must be protected, but girls' sexuality. It is up to women to redeem their moral inferiors, the men who sexually exploit them. Men are the subject of particular sexual appetites that they cannot control and it is up to women not to entice them. Young girls must be prepared for this role from birth. Within this context the innocent childhood pose is not just there to protect the child, but to control man's impulsive behaviour. Unfortunately, it also contributes towards fetishes about innocence and virginity. Thus the sexually provocative pose suggest that the child is somehow 'asking for it' and is not a victim of adult power.

Media scandals

One hundred and fifty years of the child-rearing expert has provided many contradictions. Are children an almost infinitely flexible receptacle of specific socialisation practices; a seething mass of unconscious sexuality and aggression; or elaborated puppies undergoing house-training (Rogers, 1993)? Does masturbation cause untold physical and psychological damage or is it harmless? Are mother's to blame or is mother-blaming a patriarchal conspiracy? While the propaganda of the child-rearing expert has covered the pages of respectable journals, dedicated to the pursuit of truth through scientific research, it has been left to the media to expose the scandals that exist in the world of childhood sexuality and to publish the research that society is more reluctant to accept. In February 1996, *The Guardian* related the findings of a study called 'The Game's Up', the Children's Society pointed out that child prostitutes do not seem to be labelled sexually abused. In 1992, of 3000 children known to be working in the sex trade, only 253 men were charged with unlawful sexual intercourse with a girl under 13 years (Kane, 1996). The majority of this number were men abusing children in the home, eg. a stepfather. However, between 1989 and 1993, 3300 children below the age of 18 years were charged or convicted of sexual offences. This gives a very clear message that the girls are to blame.

Begging and prostitution are the only prospects for many young people because of mass unemployment (Gayton, 1993). This echoes the discourse on sexuality in general and prostitution in particular in the nineteenth century. It appears that when society is undergoing rapid change and work possibilities are limited, moral panics are generated. If society is in decline, control must be exercised, particularly over the working-class and by the state if necessary.

Newspaper reports also covered the British diplomat who was convicted for illegally importing paedophile videos and, from time to time, report on seemingly isolated cases of sexual assault in children's homes, including a report into a Birmingham council that suppressed findings about teenage prostitution where at least 20 girls were thought to be at risk (Anon, *Observer*, 1995). The greatest outrage, however, is reserved for the exploitation of children in Thailand and the Philippines where holidays are organised for men which include sex with children. These activities are condemned with the greatest moral outrage whereas reports in Great Britain are criticised for exaggerating the problems.

The secret suffering of children

The secret suffering of children is revealed quite poignantly in the statistics generated by the counsellors at Childline (Neustatter, 1996). Childline set up ten years ago as a free confidential help-line receives 10 000 calls a day, although the five regional centres with 750 counsellors can only deal with about a third of them. The sad indictment of 150 years of child-rearing experts' advice is that when adults are presumed to know best, it is difficult for children to believe they have the right to speak out. Adults have a vested interest in maintaining some of the myths otherwise a failure of monumental proportions must be admitted. Politicians need to maintain control over what they see as declining morality and cannot hold themselves responsible. So they must blame a group of individuals in which the morality of society has been invested for over 100 years — the family. We want our child abusers to be deviants out there on the margins, few in number, frightened, deformed creatures, not figures of power and authority, smiling with their public faces, and not so many of them (Grant, 1996). Esther Rantzen's Childwatch did not uncover the truth about child sexual abuse, it made public what some professionals and some feminist activists knew already. The most startling fact in Childwatch's specially commissioned opinion poll was not: that four out of five children felt they could not tell any one about their abuse; that of the one in five who did tell, 75% said it did no good or that because of lack of evidence only 15% of those cases ever went to court, but that nine out of ten children suffering abuse were abused by members of their own family. Despite the concerns over the taboo of incest that underpinned Freud's original ideas about the dynamic unconscious; despite the revolution in house design to avoid the sexual promiscuity that might arise from overcrowding as advocated by Beatrice Webb when working for Booth in 1888; despite the laws that make it illegal, incest is an integral part of the fabric of our society (Wohl, 1978). The child prostitute, the paedophile, the sexually-abused, the pregnant adolescent is all part of the continuum that is the sexual mores of British society. Denying the extent of the problem is to perpetuate it and prevent suitable strategies evolving to overcome it. Alice Miller goes as far as to say, it is what perpetuates the violence that we see all around us. While it only appears to happen to a few; while we can categorise the Wests, the Hamiltons and the Hindleys of our world as evil, then we will not be forced to face the broad continuum of sexual perversion that is within us all. We will continue to find new ways to avoid the truth. Politicians will wrap it up in a moral panic while sex educationalists want to accept the limited evidence and plug the gap with more available contraception. The law continues to enforce some age-old rhetoric about childhood innocence. A more important strategy for future generations would be to enlighten children about healthy sexuality and encourage them to say no to all unwanted advances, just as children recently have been taught to say no to strangers in respect of road safety. The problem with this approach is that those they need to reject may be the very people from whom they should expect advice — the heart of their own families.

How can we prepare our young for adulthood and enable them to make mature decisions about pregnancy? By giving them respect, particularly for their differences, allowing them gradually increasing independence, providing them with relevant information, support and an unambiguous declaration and clarification of their civil status. Most importantly, we should offer protection for all the vulnerable, not just 'deserving individuals' whose selection is based on historically constructed, patriarchal interpretations of sexuality that denies childhood sexuality in order to maintain adult control, but a full recognition of the power relations in sexuality from childhood to maturity. This will involve recognition of all deviant forms of sexuality: child abuse, prostitution, paedophillia and adolescent pregnancy, as part of a continuum of the same problem.

Broken images

Politicians and child health experts are confident that the evidence produces clear images about the causes of adolescent pregnancy. I have argued that these are fractured and incomplete. In emphasising the relationship between sexual victimisation in childhood and its concomitant problems in adolescence and beyond, I hope I have shared a new understanding of my confusion.

'He continues quick and dull in his clear images;
I continue slow and sharp in my broken images.

He in a new confusion of his understanding;
I in a new understanding of my confusion.'

Robert Graves, 1986

References

Allen de Villbiss L (1920) The habit training of young children. *Mat Child Welfare* **IV**: 26–7

Anon (1894) The mother and her boy. *Home Notes* Aug 18th. : 158

Anon (1982) Teenage girls getting pregnant to beat the dole queue. *Daily Telegraph* December 30th

Anon (1995) In-care child sex report. *The Observer* October 15th

Ariès P (1973) *Centuries of Childhood*, 2nd edn. Penguin, Harmondsworth

Bachman G, Moeller T, Bennett J (1988) Childhood sexual abuse and the consequences in adult women. *Obstet Gynaecol* **71**: 631–41

Barrett M (1980) *Women's Oppression Today: Problems in Marxist Feminist Analysis*. Verso, London

Bass E, Davis L (1988) *The Courage to Heal: A Guide for the Survivors of Child Sexual Abuse*. Cedar, London

Bowlby J (1951) *Maternal Care and Mental Health*. Shocken Books, New York

Boyer D, Fine D (1992) Sexual abuse as a factor in adolescent pregnancy and child maltreatment. *Fam Plan Perspect* **24**: 4–11

Boyle M (1991) Decision making for contraception and abortion. In: Pitts M, Phillips K, eds. *The Psychology of Health: An Introduction*. Routledge, London

Brook Advisory Centres (1992) *Annual Report*. Walworth, London

Butler JR, Burton LM (1990) Rethinking teenage child bearing: Is sexual abuse a missing link? *Fam Relat* **39**: 73–80

Cassidy J (1995) Sex and the single mother. *Nurs Times* **91**(34): 18

Chodorow N (1978) *The Reproduction of Mothering*. University of California Press, Berkeley

Clark E (1989) *Young Single Mothers Today: A Qualitative Study of Housing and Support Needs*. National Council for One Parent Families, London

Cook R (1993) Preventing unwanted teenage pregnancies. *Nurs Stand* **7**(38): 28–30

Cook V (1995) Maternity Projects: Teenage Pregnancies. *Midwives* **108**: 76–9.

Corbin A (1990) *Women for Hire, Prostitution and Sexuality In France after 1850*. Harvard University Press, London

Cvetkovich G, Grote B (1981) Psychosocial maturity and teenage contraceptive use: An investigation of decision making and communication skills. *Pop Environ* **4**: 211–26

Dellacoste F, Alexander P, eds. (1987) *Sex Work: Writings by Women in the Industry*. Cleis Press, Pittsburgh

Department of Health (1992) *The Health of the Nation*. HMSO, London

Doherty S (1995) Single mothers: A critical issue. *Fem Psychol* **5**(1):105–11

Ellis H (1936) *Studies in the Psychology of Sex*, vol 1, part 2. The Sexual Impulse in Women. Random House, New York

Family Planning Association (1980) *Bristol Booking Survey*. FPA, London

Finkelhor D (1986) *A Source Book on Child Sexual Abuse*. Sage, Beverly Hills

Firestone S (1979) The Dialectic of Sex: The Case for Feminist Revolution. Women's Press, London

Foucault M (1979) The History of Sexuality, vol 1. An introduction. Allen Lane, London. Cited in: Weeks J (1989) *Sex, Politics and Society*, 2nd edn. Longman, London

Freud S (1940) *An Outline of Psychoanalysis*. Translation Strachey J (1969) Hogarth Press, London

Freud S (1977) Three essays on the theory of sexuality. In: *On Sexuality*. Pelican Freud Library, vol 7, Harmondsworth

Furstenberg FF, Lincoln R, Menken J (1981) *Teenage Sexuality and Child Bearing*. University of Pennsylvania Press, Philadelphia

Gayton R (1993) Begging and prostitution. *The Guardian*, **June 16**: 5

Gershenson HP, Musick JS, Ruch-Ross HS, Magee V, Rubino KK, Rosenberg D (1989) The prevalence of coercive sexual experience among teenage mothers. *J Interpers Viol* **4**: 204–19

Gillick v West Norfolk Health Authority (1986) AC 112, (10985) 3 A11 ER 402, (1985 3 JOUR 830)

Grant L (1996) Beyond Belief. *The Guardian*, **Sep 14th** : 22 –8

Graves R (1986) In: O'Prey P, ed. *Selected Poems*. Penguin, Harmondsworth

Hollway W (1989) *Subjectivity and Method in Psychology : Gender, Meaning and Science*. Sage, London

Howard M, cited in Waterhouse R (1993) Family values: single mothers — how many are there? *Independent on Sunday*, **Nov 14th**: 11

Hutter B, Williams G (1981) Controlling women: The normal and the deviant. In: Hutter B, Williams G, eds. *Controlling Women: The Normal and the Deviant*. Croom Helm, London

Kane M (1996) Death of innocence. *The Guardian*, **Feb 12th** (Guardian 2: 2)

Key E (1909) *The Century of the Child*. Logos, Uppsala

King C (1992) The politics of representation: A democracy of the gaze. In: Bonner F, Goodman L, Allen R, Jones L, King C, eds. *Imagining*

Women's Cultural Representations and Gender. Polity Press, Cambridge

Kirby H (1989) How old is old enough? *The Times*, **Sep 11th**, 19

Kuhn A (1980) Remembrance. In: Spence J, Holland P (1991) *Family Snaps. The Meaning of Domestic Photography*. Virago, London

Lanz JB (1995) Psychological, behavioural, and social characteristics associated with early forced sexual intercourse among pregnant adolescents. *J Interpers Viol* **10**(2): 188–200

Littlejohn P (1992) Teenage pregnancy and adolescent motherhood in Australia: Research in progress. Cited in: Moore S, Rosenthal D (1993) *Sexuality in Adolescence*. Routledge, London

Luker K (1975) *Taking Chances: Abortion and the Decision not to Contracept*. University of California Press, Berkeley

Luker K (1977) Contraceptive risk-taking and abortion: results and implications of a San Francisco Bay study. *Stud Fam Plan* **8** : 190–6

Makinson, C (1985) Young age per se does not make a high risk pregnancy. *Fam Plan Perspect* **17**: 13

Mander G (1996) The stifled cry or Truby King, the forgotten prophet. Br J Psychother 13(1): ??page nos??

Mann S (1991) *Immediate Family*. Phaidon Press, London

Marcus S (1967) The other Victorians: A study of sexuality and pornography in mid-nineteenth century England. Weidenfield and Nicholson, London. Cited in: Weeks J (1989) *Sex, Politics and Society*, 2nd edn. Longman, Harlow

Marot F (1994) Teenagers and sex: a suitable case for education. *Prof Care Mother Child* **4**(2): 46–8

De Mause L, ed. (1974) *The History of Childhood*. The Psychohistory Press, New York

McMahon M (1991) Nursing histories reviving life in abandoned selves. *Fem Rev* **37**: 23–37

Miller A (1992) *Breaking Down the Wall of Silence to Join the Waiting Child*. Virago, London

Mills JG (1988) Survey of teenage attitudes to pregnancy within the Northern district of Glasgow. *Midwives Chron Nurs Notes* **101**(1207): 243–5

Moore S (1992) The real embarrassment of riches. *The Guardian* **Oct 1st** : 19

Morrison DM (1985) Adolescent contraceptive behaviour: A review. *Psycholog Bull* **98**: 538–68

Neustatter A (1996) Ten years on, the late night calls still break our hearts. You, *The Mail on Sunday* **27th Oct**: 34–5

Oakley A (1981) *From Here to Maternity*. Penguin, Harmondsworth

Paterson A. *George Eliot's Life and Letters*, vol 1. Selwyn and Blount, London

Phoenix A (1993) The social construction of teenage motherhood: A Black and White issue? In: Lawson A, Rhode DL, eds. *The Politics of Pregnancy*. Yale University Press, London

Prendergast S, Prout A (1980) What will I do... ? Teenage girls and the construction of motherhood. *Sociolog Rev* **8**: 517

Proust M (1984) *Swann's Way. Book One of Remembrance of Things Past. Penguin*, London

Rainey DY, Stevens-Simons C, Kaplan DW (1995) Are adolescents who report prior sexual abuse at higher risk for pregnancy? *Child Abuse Neg* **19**(10): 1283–8

Ranjan V (1993) Pregnancy in the under-16s: waking up to the realities. *Prof Care Mother Child* **3**(2): 34–5

Rogers RS (1993) The social construction of child-rearing. In: Beatie A, Gott M, Jones L, Sidell M, eds. *Health and Well-being: A Reader*. Macmillan, Open University Press, Basingstoke

Rousseau JJ (1762) *Émile*, 1963 edn. Dent, London

Royal College of Obstetricians and Gynaecologists (1991) *Report of the RCOG Working Party on Unplanned Pregnancy*. RCOG, London

Russell B (1946) *The History of Western Philosophy*. George Allen and Unwin, London

Russell DEH (1983) The incidence and prevalence of intrafamilial and extrafamilial abuse of female children. *Child Abuse Neg* **7**: 133–46

Sayer J (1982) *Biological Politics*. Tavistock, London

Scally G (1992) Teenage pregnancy: The challenge of prevention, Sir William Power Memorial Lecture. *Midwives Chron* **106**(1226): 232–9

Spence J, Holland P (1991) *Family Snaps. The Meanings of Domestic Photography*. Virago, London

Spock B (1979) *Baby and Childcare*, 4 edn. Bodley Head, London

Stevens-Simons C, Reichert S (1994) Sexual abuse, adolescent pregnancy, and child abuse. A developmental approach to an intergenerational cycle. *Arch Pediatr Adolesc Health* **148**: 23–7

Stone L (1981) Children and the family. In: Barnes P, Oates J, Chapman J, Lee V, Czerniewska P, eds. *Personality Development and Learning*. Hoddor and Stoughton, London: 8–17

Tong R (1989) *Feminist Thought: A Comprehensive Introduction*. Routledge, London

Warner M (1994) *Six Myths of Our Time: Managing Monsters*. Vintage, London

Watson JB (1928) *Psychological Care of the Infant and Child*. W W Norton, New York. Reprinted in 1972 by Arno Press, New York

Weeks J (1989) *Sex, Politics and Society*, 2nd edn. Longman, Harlow

Wegner DM, Vallacher RR (1977) *Implicit Psychology: An Introduction to Social Cognition*. Oxford University Press, Oxford

Whyatt GE (1985) The sexual abuse of Afro-American and white American women in childhood. *Child Abuse Neg* **9**: 507–19

Williams V (1992) The naked truth. *The Guardian,* **Sept 22nd**: 17

Wohl AS (1978) Sex and the single room: Incest among the Victorian working classes. In: Wohl AS, ed. *The Victorian Family*. Croom Helm, London

8
Health and people with learning disabilities

Tony Gilbert

The sexuality of people with learning disabilities is, and has been, a problematic area in health and social welfare policy and practice since the early nineteenth century. This chapter aims to construct a discussion that links the development of ideas in this particular section of the population, with the development of ideas about sexuality. This may appear to be a rather abstract approach to sexual health. However, it is the contention here that, to appreciate the context within which practice takes place, a clear understanding of how that context comes to be formed is required.

The world of people with learning disabilities is haunted by contradictory ideas of the innocent and the dangerous (Williams, 1992). These ideas, once overtly stated in public debates and policy, are now covert (Brown, 1994). The dangerous, feeble-minded and morally defective who concerned the philanthropists and eugenicists of the Victorian period come to be redefined in the more liberal discourses of the second half of the twentieth century. Here the sexuality and the sex education of people with learning disabilities are seen as key issues in professional discussions of correct practice.

However, we must be careful not to fall too easily into the trap of seeing this change as evolutionary, taking us from the dark ages of Victorian repression to some form of enlightenment. Rather, we need to consider how the interplay of a variety of discourses of care and control come together at particular moments to produce historically, specific categorisations and their related mechanisms of social control. Indeed, 'learning disability' is merely the latest in a series of categorisations, developed through the classification by the professions of medicine, law, education and psychology, of people who were seen to have failed to meet various norms relating to intellectual functioning. Previous categorisations include: the nineteenth and early twentieth century notions of idiot, imbecile, feeble-minded and morally defective, the mid-twentieth century notion of the mentally subnormal, and later twentieth century notions of the mentally-handicapped or retarded.

There is also a danger of seeing people with learning disabilities as a homogeneous group. Hilary Brown (1994) points to how these contradictory ideas of innocence and the dangerous could be found within the same services promoting different practices for people with different levels of learning disability. She describes how one hospital ward contained only men, the rationale being their potential for sexual behaviour, while on a neighbouring ward, men and women with multiple disabilities slept in the same dormitories, the rationale being that they were asexual. These issues are developed in the following section.

Biological or social: the problem of sexuality

Jeffery Weeks (1981) identifies a central question which lays at the heart of discussions of sexuality and, by implication, questions of sexual health. 'Should sexuality be seen as the result of powerful biological and instinctual forces which shape the individual and the institutions of the social world, and where repression of this force leads to some form of ill health such as neurosis or perversion?' This, 'essentialist', position holds a powerful influence. However, it has been challenged by those who have argued that sexuality is the product of social and cultural moulding. This latter position maintains that nothing is intrinsically sexual, or alternatively, anything can be sexualised. This position is expressed most forcibly in the work of Michel Foucault (1980), who describes sexuality as a historical apparatus through which sex is regulated and controlled, and through which various 'experts' deploy their discourses of normality.

These two positions, 'essentialist' versus 'social constructionalist', provide quite different strategies for intervention, although they may draw upon similar human technologies, eg. teaching techniques, counselling. For this reason it is essential to establish the nature of the discourses which underlie particular practices. The 'essentialist' position poses questions on how, and in what way, this instinctual force can be safely and healthily channelled or contained. Many of the present day attitudes and practices relating to sexuality and people with learning disabilities can be located within this position. Here apparently contradictory discourses coexist. This results in both the denial of sexuality and the training of people in what are considered to be appropriate and normal sexual behaviours.

The 'social constructionalist' position raises a set of different questions. These relate to the historical processes through which both gender and sexuality have come to be defined in their present form. These should be woven into the processes of definition that have produced the label 'learning disabled.' There are two general effects of this process of classification and categorisation. The first is to separate a particular group of people from the general population and the second distinguishes this group from other groups who have been given a different category and segregation. These segregated groups are then compared to particular sets of norms and marked as different (Foucault, 1979).

Foucault argues that the development of discourses of sexuality in the late nineteenth and early twentieth century focused upon four issues: the hysterisation of women's bodies, a pedagogisation of children's sex, a socialisation of procreative behaviours and the psychiatrisation of perverse pleasures. These in turn produced four categories of person for investigation and regulation: the hysterical woman, the masturbating child, the Malthusian couple and the perverse adult (Foucault, 1980).

These categories are of particular interest to this discussion. The hysterical woman was in danger of producing defective children; the masturbating child was in danger of compromising his intellectual and moral health and, therefore, undermining his line of descent; the Malthusian couple engaged in unrestrained reproduction and were the source of the unfit; and the perverse adult was both the target and the promoter of all forms of immorality and vice. The influence of these categories has impacted upon the lives of the population, especially upon the lives of people with learning disabilities, and can be identified within present day practices. From this position of 'social construction' the 'essentialist' claim is not rejected as such, rather its status as a form of truth is challenged, and it is identified as the result of a particular configuration of ideas (Foucault, 1980).

The discussion of sexual health and people with learning disability requires a recognition of the social and historical process which comes to define sexuality, gender and learning disability. This is because people with learning disabilities are gendered and they may, at points in their lives, express themselves as heterosexual, bisexual or homosexual. They may also participate in a range of implicit or explicit sexual practices. Finally, as Williams points out, 'However, what is particularly significant for women who have learning difficulties is that many of the stereotypes about people with learning difficulties converge with sexist and racist stereotyping' (Williams, 1992), a comment which has some validity when applied to men with learning disabilities.

This route is complex. It has its roots in the production of techniques for the management of the population from the eighteenth century onwards and is located within the social construction of family life. Moreover, it has to consider the effects of pathologising non-reproductive sexual activity upon people with learning disabilities and on others without learning disabilities. This leads to a discussion of the emergence of different sexual identities and the relationship between sexual identity and sexual health.

Managing the population: the feeble-minded and sexual perverts

Weeks (1981) notes that the management of the population, which had been a concern since the eighteenth century, came to be seen in the late nineteenth and early twentieth centuries as the key to national wealth and power. This debate, raising questions of national decline, unemployment, poverty and threats of war, became a debate over sex, 'And sex was the key to the question of the population. It was the point of access both to the health and status of the individual and to the future of the population as a whole' (Weeks 1985a). These issues were as- sociated with the Malthusian fear that the poor and unfit would engage in reckless over-breeding.

Degeneration was the concern of the respectable classes and morality, the key to halting the decline. These concerns were central to the emerging eugenics movement and its theory of heredity, and to the reforming zeal of campaigners, such as Charles Booth and the Fabian, Sidney Webb. Weeks (1985a) notes that sexual variations came to be associated with the key problem of poverty, 'Dr. Rentoul of Liverpool, one of the more extreme eugenicists, could easily lump together lunatics, neurotics, kleptomaniacs, alcoholics and sexual perverts as all being examples of degenerate stock.' (Weeks 1985a). While Sir Francis Galton spoke of the need to arrest a 'very serious and growing danger to our national efficiency in the growth of the feeble-minded'. Weeks (1981) also notes the way in which the population and issues relating to family life — the conditions for reproduction, were central to the formation and development of the welfare state from the 1940s onwards.

The key issue here is that these population debates linked people with learning disabilities and people who engaged in a range of non-reproductive sexual practices. Both groups were seen as challenging the heterosexual norm and, therefore, failing to conform to middle-class ideas of moral respectability. The consequence was that they became the subject matter of the emerging 'sciences' of the population (medicine, psychiatry, sexology, sociology and psychology). These 'knowledges' then produced rationales for the targeting of such groups for social surveillance and their subjection to techniques of normalisation (Foucault, 1979).

Constructing gender: constructing sexuality

Jeffrey Weeks describes a powerful central theme in essentialist discussions of sexuality. This is the linking of ideas about what constitutes normal behaviour to assumptions over what is natural. This is especially so in the case of biological sex and assumptions over gender roles. 'Conceptions about the inherent 'natural' basis of the separate social roles of men and women, and of the relationship between these roles and sexual behaviour, are deeply rooted and, far from being undermined, were actually reinforced by post-Darwinian speculation' (Weeks 1981). These natural roles, male participation in the public world of work and female involvement in domestic activity and procreation, are linked with a particular conception of the family.

The patriarchal, heterosexual, nuclear family provides a powerful ideological norm against which all forms of interpersonal relationships are compared, 'As sexuality is increasingly privatised, seen as the characteristic of the private sphere, as its public manifestations are challenged (in terms that speak all the time of sex while denying it), so deviant forms of sex become subject to more closely defined public regulation. The family norm is strengthened by a series of extramarital regulations, which refer back at all times to its normality and morality. This is, of course, underlined by a whole series of other developments, from the enforcement of the Poor Laws and the factory acts to the welfare state support of particular household models in the twentieth century' (Weeks 1991).

Underlying these assumptions about natural roles is a conception of sexuality as basically male. Females are seen as innocent, with their sexuality limited to the 'natural' desire to conceive (Weeks, 1981). This has major implications for sexuality as it becomes linked to both moral and eugenic discourses. Here, non-reproductive sexual practices, even those between married couples, come to be seen as both immoral and undesirable as they frustrate the aim of sexual activity — reproduction (Weeks, 1991). These discourses work in such a way that people with learning disabilities can find themselves excluded from these 'natural' social roles of males and females, and from sexual relations. In the case of social roles, employment (Wertheimer, 1981; Jenkins, 1989) and childcare are often denied to people with learning disabilities (Williams, 1992). At the same time, eugenic themes of the racially unfit preclude sexual relationships for the purpose of procreation, while moral themes work to exclude the possibility of non-reproductive forms of sexual activity (Walkowitz, 1985; Weeks, 1991).

Williams links the position of women with learning disabilities to that of women in general. She is especially concerned with the role women play in caring for others, both formally and informally. She argues that, while motherhood itself is denied to the majority of women with learning disabilities, caring is an important aspect of many of these women's lives, 'However, in their cases, it is caring as daughters and sisters, occasionally as wives, but rarely as mothers' (Williams, 1992). Williams goes on to point out that these expectations of domestic labour appear to obstruct admittance into the public world of paid employment. Instead it cements the position of these women into the private world of domestic labour.

A consequence of this is that women with learning disabilities find their lives being constricted to a greater degree than men with learning disabilities, with less opportunities for social experiences or independent living. Williams also notes the lack of support for women with learning disabilities in acquiring competence in personal care in areas such as menstruation. Similarly, Clements *et al* (1995), note the absence in the literature of issues relating to women with learning disabilities and the menopause. The position of women with learning disabilities in having their gender constrained by the denial of both motherhood and paid employment, can be contrasted with the social construction of femininity where pronatalist values hold the role of the mother in high esteem (Riley, 1985).

This, in turn, can be contrasted with the social construction of masculinity. Patriarchal authority is derived from the public world, in part through paid employment and in part through the embedding of the 'male world view' in the social institutions of contemporary western society. The social position of men with a learning disability is seen to be derived through these same gendered power relations. In welfare services, patriarchal values are seen to dominate, with needs set in terms of the 'individual' and responses linked to scientific 'technologies', such as medicine and psychology. Feminine values relating to communication, relationships and emotion are subjugated (Clements *et al*, 1995). This places women with learning disabilities at a double disadvantage. Firstly, their potential for motherhood is denied and, secondly, their needs are subjected to a male interpretation.

However, there is a tendency to assume that there is less tension between the gender roles of men generally and those of men with learning disabilities. Williams (1992) points to the greater freedom enjoyed by men with learning disabilities, while Clements *et al* note that role models within services tend to reinforce patriarchal structures in the way males tend to dominate in positions of authority and women tend to play subordinate roles, 'People with learning disabilities often have very limited social opportunities and the interactions of staff provide very powerful role models for them. The kinds of gender-based divisions outlined above will compound the oppression of the women who use the service and will encourage the men to see women as of less consequence, and to see relationships as primarily about power' (Clements *et al*, 1995).

The problem with this assumption is that it ignores the real tensions that exist between the position of men with learning disabilities and the social construction of masculinity. In patriarchal relations there is no social role accorded to men which does not revolve around participation in the public sphere. The tasks of work, of defence and of politics are ideologically male, despite increasing female participation. Men with learning disabilities experience exclusion from all of these. The basis of male power, which tends to be physical and financial (Williams and Watson, 1988), is also far more tentative when viewed in the context of men with learning disabilities. The increased incidence of physical and sensory disabilities in people with learning disability (Department of Health, 1995) means that physical strength is less likely to provide a basis for power, while the problem of access to employment and reliance upon benefits means that many people with learning disability experience poverty (Sumpton, 1988; Jenkins, 1989), thus negating the basis for economic power.

There is also the problem of fatherhood. Women with learning disabilities who become mothers may be seen as vulnerable or immoral, but men with learning disabilities who become fathers are more likely to be seen as dangerous. Essentialist discourse considers male sexual desire to be in need of strict self-control (Weeks, 1981). Public displays of procreative ability by men with learning disabilities are likely to be linked with the idea of the perverse adult. Brown (1994) indicates that the language, which has been used in contemporary scientific discourse concerning people with learning disabilities, has paralleled that used until recently against homosexuals, ie. sick, immature or perverted.

At the same time, Heyman and Huckle (1995) suggest that sexuality is perceived as a hazard in the lives of people with learning disabilities. They identify how some informal carers saw sexuality to be a source of danger to be avoided. Carers feared that sexual knowledge could lead to the male person sexually abusing others or the female person becoming pregnant. The issue of whether such knowledge helps the person with learning disabilities to resist being abused is avoided, this despite the growing evidence of the vulnerability of people with learning disabilities (Brown and Craft, 1989; Sinason, 1994; Sobsey, 1994). The problem of masculinity and learning disability can also be seen in the context of fatherhood. Tymchuk and Andron (1996) point to the fact that most research relating to parenthood and people with learning disabilities is focused upon the mothers. There is little focus upon the fathers of the children or upon the current partners of these women. Booth and Booth (1994) observe a similar exclusion of fathers in their work with parents with a learning disability.

The ambiguities in responses to gender issues are not made any easier through the support offered to people with learning disabilities. Clements *et al* argue that there is a tendency in welfare services, upon which many people with learning disabilities rely, towards gender blindness. This ignoring of gender differences is compounded by a sexuality blindness. This, they argue, functions as a process of censorship in the lives of people with a learning disability. However, the liberal discourse of contemporary practice demands a more sophisticated response than the simple segregation practised in the mental deficiency colonies of old, 'Ultimately, many staff would be more comfortable if they did not have 'it' but if a politically correct response is required, then people with learning disabilities should be taught very clearly about meaningful relationships; not getting pregnant and not getting AIDS. Important though these things are — where is the fun, where is the sex as it is known and experienced by at least some real men and real women, be they lesbian, gay, bisexual or heterosexual' (Clements *et al*, 1995).

Sexuality, pleasure and identity

The discussion of sexual health has to go beyond discussions of technique and protection. It has to raise questions concerning; who we are and who we identify with, whether we experience oppression in this identification and in who or what do we find pleasure. For people with learning disabilities, these questions raise issues of power relating to choice, opportunity and privacy. Therefore, the discussion of sexuality and sexual health has to take place within the context of relationships, but what is the nature of these relationships?

Giddens (1991) claims that, as 'Modernity' has given way to 'High Modernity', traditional forms of living have given way to a diversity of choices. This has brought with it anxiety and uncertainty, which threatens self-identity. Moreover, the choice of 'lifestyle' has become central to the structuring of self-identity. Intimacy, which is at the heart of modern forms of friendship and established sexual relationships, becomes the quest for individuals. This requires psychological work and is only possible between individuals who are secure in their own self-identity. Giddens continues by pointing out that this requires commitment and the sharing of a meaningful lifestyle.

Weeks (1981; 1985b; 1991) offers a thorough discussion of sexual identity developed in the social and historical context of both male and female sexuality. This provides the basis for a discussion of sexual identity in people with learning disabilities. Weeks argues that identity is both fragile, through incessant challenges from social contingencies and psychic demands, and necessary, as it provides the foundation of our sexual beliefs and behaviours. He argues that the idea of sexual identity should not be taken lightly, 'For many in the modern world — especially the sexually marginal — it is an absolutely fundamental concept, offering a sense of personal unity, social location and even, at times, a political commitment' (Weeks, 1991).

This raises a number of issues in relation to people with learning disabilities for, as we have seen, they are in danger of being sexually marginalised. Questions of lifestyle choice, of homosexuality and lesbianism or of heterosexuality, are set within welfare services which operate within the implicit notion of the 'naturalness' of the nuclear family (Muncie and Wetherall, 1993). Against this, Weeks (1981; 1991) notes the development, from the eighteenth century onwards, for the medical and legal prescription of normality and the boundaries of the erotic to address a tendency to view sexual practices, not in terms of acts, but in terms of the personality characteristics of the actor. Weeks locates the counter movement to the categorisation of sexual practices, which fail to conform to the heterosexual norm, as perverse, with the development in the 1950s of liberal views linking identity with individualism. Movements of 'resistance' have formed in places, such as San Francisco, producing communities of the sexually-marginalised, 'Women and men have mobilised around their sense of sexual identity in such a place because it was in their sexuality that they felt most powerfully invalidated' (Weeks 1991).

However, the relationship between sexual identity and sexual practice is complex for, as Weeks notes, there is no necessary connection between the two, 'Sexual identity is a strange thing. There are some people who identify as gay and participate in the gay community but do not experience or wish for homosexual activity. And there are many homosexually active people who do not identify as gay. Many black homosexuals, for example, prefer to identify with black rather than gay political positions' (Weeks 1991). At this point, it is worth noting that celibacy can be a lifestyle choice for some people regardless of their sexual orientation. This does not compromise their sexual identity. Therefore, this has to be kept distinct from ideas of people with learning disabilities as asexual.

This contradiction of sexual identity and sexual practice can be most clearly seen in the case of lesbianism. Weeks points out that the construction of lesbianism by sexologists as a sexual category has been challenged by feminists, 'Among gay men the issue has fundamentally concerned sex, validating a denied sexuality. In debates on lesbianism, on the other hand, there have been heated exchanges about the necessary connection of a lesbian identity to sexual practices' (Weeks, 1991). Lesbianism, in contrast to male homosexuality, has not been linked to casual anonymous sex. Rather, it is described as a profoundly female experience based in women's emotion and affection for each other, and in the rejection of male tyranny (Weeks, 1991).

The question of relationships (number, type and quality) is, therefore, critical to the sexual health of people with learning disabilities as they provide the very basis for identity. Clements *et al* note the difficulties for people with learning disabilities, 'For lesbians and gay men with learning disabilities the problem is exacerbated by the lack of acknowledgement and understanding of their chosen sexuality and their lack of access to the gay and lesbian community. If service users are brave enough to assert their sexuality, they may be lucky enough to have it acknowledged; and, if it is, they can have their desires interpreted — at best as 'uninformed' or 'indiscriminate', or at worst as 'abnormal' or 'perverted'.' (Clements *et al*, 1995). The identification with a particular community, whether it be heterosexual, homosexual, or related to race and culture, is a particular problem for many people with learning disabilities. This may be due to social isolation (Chappell, 1992), to the attitudes of informal and formal carers (Heyman and Huckle, 1995: Clements *et al*, 1995), or to the imposition of simplistic sexual models in services (Brown, 1994).

It might be argued that the link between perceptions of people with learning disabilities as innocent or dangerous lies in relationships. Innocence is set in a condition where there are no relationships. There is no identity, no potential for sexual activity, no desire, no risk. On the other hand, dangerousness increases as relationships develop. They provide the basis for identity, especially sexual identity, and carry with them the danger of stimulating sexual desire.

This concern over relationships can be seen in a study by Heyman and Huckle (1995). The assertion of a sexual identity, albeit in heterosexual terms, was perceived by carers to be a hazard. Responses include: prohibition, anxiety over ability to manage relationships and fears of abuse or of the person abusing. Interestingly, this study suggested that people with learning disabilities have quite conservative attitudes towards sexual relations within their personal relationships. However, the relationships were very important to the people involved. Heyman and Huckle note that this may be a consequence of the attitude of the carers, but these difficulties are not limited only to the perspectives of carers.

In the context of what might be described as the supreme assertion of heterosexual identity — parenting, Booth and Booth (1994) describe the experiences of a number of parents with learning disabilities. They describe the struggle to survive in a hostile environment characterised by poverty, the negative attitudes of child protection workers and the unsupportive responses of social welfare services. Again, this study suggests that persons with learning disabilities take their personal relationships very seriously, but have quite conservative attitudes towards sexual relationships. The study also proposes that these relationships, like all relationships, are dynamic with some changes resulting in breaking up.

Finally, there is the issue of pleasure. Clements *et al* (1995) note that in the lives of real men and real women sex was fun. However, the idea of pleasure is often omitted from discussions of sexuality and people with learning disabilities, and personal relationships are reduced to notions of appropriate behaviour and techniques. There are a wide range of practices, which are seen to provide pleasure and many of these involve close and intimate contact with other people, especially people in whom one has a degree of personal trust. These may include food and drink, or forms of intimate touch. Or these activities may be highly individual in their association with pleasure, bearing in mind Foucault's point that a range of activities can become sexualised (Foucault, 1980).

The problems of privacy experienced by many people with learning disabilities, means that there is a danger that some sexualised practices may be interpreted as perverse, or as 'challenging behaviours', which services then seek to prohibit. There is also the issue, highlighted by Brown and Barrett (1994), that a lack of opportunities may constrict the development of sexual practices leaving the individual with obsessive sexual rituals.

Summary

This discussion of sexual health and people with learning disabilities reaches three basic conclusions. The first is that, when working with this section of society, approaches to sexual health have to be informed by an appreciation of how their sexuality has been and continues to be marginalised. Secondly, the issue of identity has to be central to any approach. This requires an understanding of the ways in which both gender identity and sexual identity are formed, and of the contradictions and tensions which may exist between these. The third relates to the context. Many people with learning disabilities rely upon the support of welfare services. In many cases these services offer little in the way of privacy, while, at the same time, maintaining a close surveillance of people's activities. This can lead to the interpretation of sexual activity as perverse, with attempts at prohibition.

References

Booth T, Booth W (1994) *Parenting Under Pressure: Mothers and Fathers with Learning Difficulties*. Open University Press, Milton Keynes

Brown H, Craft A (1989) *Thinking the Unthinkable: Papers on Sexual Abuse and People with Learning Difficulties*. Family Planning Association, London.

Brown H (1994) An ordinary sexual life: a review of the normalisation principle as it applies to the sexual options of people with learning disabilities. *Disabil Soc* **9**(2): 123–43

Brown H, Barrett S (1994) Understanding and responding to difficult sexual behaviour. In: Craft A, ed. *Practice Issues in Sexuality and Learning Disabilities*. Routledge, London: 50–80

Chappell AL (1992) Towards a sociological critique of the normalisation principle. *Disabil Handicap Soc* **7**(1): 35–51

Clements J, Clare I, Ezelle LA (1995) Real men, real women, real lives? Gender issues in learning disabilities and challenging behaviour. *Disabil Soc* **10**(4): 425–35

Department of Health (1995) *The Health of the Nation: A Strategy for People with Learning Disabilities*. HMSO, London

Foucault M (1979) *Discipline and Punish: The Birth of the Prison*. Vintage/Random House, New York

Foucault M (1980) *The History of Sexuality*: vol 1, An Introduction. Vintage/Random House, New York

Giddens A (1991) *Modernity and Self-Identity: Self and Society in the Late Modern Age*. Polity Press, Cambridge

Heyman B, Huckle S (1995) Sexuality as a perceived hazard in the lives of adults with learning difficulties. *Disabil Soc* **10**(2): 139–55

Jenkins R (1989) Barriers to adulthood: Long-term unemployment and mental handicap compared. In: Brechin A, Walmsley J, eds. *Making Connections: Reflecting on the Lives and Experiences of People with Learning Difficulties*. Hodder and Stoughton, Sevenoaks: 100–8

Muncie J, Wetherall M (1993) Family policy and political discourse. In: Cochrane A, Muncie J, eds. *Politics, Policy and the Law*. Open University Press, Milton Keynes: 33–80

Riley D (1985) Post-war pronatalism. In: Beechey V, Donald J, eds. *Subjectivity and Social Relations*. Open University Press, Milton Keynes: 132–46

Sinason V (1994) Working with sexually abused individuals who have a learning disability. In: Craft A, ed. *Practice Issues in Sexuality and Learning Disabilities*. Routledge, London: 156–75.

Sobsey D (1994) Sexual Abuse of Individuals with Intellectual Disability. In: Craft A, ed. *Practice Issues in Sexuality and Learning Disabilities*. Routledge, London: 93–115.

Sumpton R (1988) Poverty and Mental Handicap. In: Becker S, MacPherson S, eds. *Public Issues, Private Pain: Poverty, Social Work and Social Policy*. Social Services Insight, London: 162–70.

Tymchuk A, Andron L (1996) Rationale, approaches, results and resource implications of programmes to enhance parenting skills of people with learning disabilities. In: Craft A, ed. *Practice Issues in Sexuality and Learning Disabilities*. Routledge, London: 202–16.

Walkowitz J (1985) Male vice and feminist virtue: Male vice and the politics of prostitution in nineteenth century Britain. In: Beechey V, Donald J, eds. *Subjectivity and Social Relations*. Open University Press, Milton Keynes: 175–88

Weeks J (1981) *Sex Politics and Society: The Regulation of Sexuality since 1800*. Longman, Edinburgh

Weeks J (1985a) The population question in the early twentieth century. In: Beechey V, Donald J, eds. *Subjectivity and Social Relations*. Open University Press, Milton Keynes: 189–201

Weeks J (1985b) *Sexuality and its Discontents: Meanings, Myths and Modern Sexualities*. Routledge and Kegan Paul, London

Weeks J (1991) *Against Nature: Essays on History, Sexuality and Identity*. Rivers Orem Press, London

Wertheimer A (1981) Disability and income. In: Walker A, Townsend P, eds. *Disability in Britain*. Martin Robertson, Oxford: 156–74

Williams F (1992) Women with learning disabilities are women too. In: Langan M, Day L, eds. *Women, Oppression and Social Work*. Routledge, London: 149–68

Williams J, Watson G (1988) Sexual inequality, family life and family therapy. In: Street E, Dryden W, eds. *Family Therapy in Britain*. Open University Press, Milton Keynes: 291–311

9
Sexuality and mental health: challenging ignorance and prejudice

Matthew V Morrissey

Sexuality for people with mental health problems is a sensitive and volatile subject which is often ignored, medicalised and avoided. This can result in dehumanising and depersonalising an integral part of human life — a person's sexuality. The stigma, ignorance and prejudicial assumptions held by many sectors of society, surrounding people with mental health problems, is compounded if their sexuality is denied. However, it is ignorant and arrogant to presume that people with mental health problems are hyposexual or have no control over their sexual drives. In this chapter, mental health and sexuality are discussed in terms of current practices, including the side-effects of medication on sexual functioning. Examples are given of problematic situations faced by hospital staff and guidelines to assess the sexual needs of people with mental health problems, eg. schizophrenia. Based on these issues, a number of recommendations will be made on ways to integrate knowledge about sexuality into practice, guided by supportive policies and structures, including users' perspectives.

Psychiatry

It is generally taboo to discuss sex with people with mental health problems, in particular with clients suffering from schizophrenia. This often leaves the client lacking in knowledge and feeling inadequate and uncertain. If psychiatry is to modernise itself as a discipline, it needs to promote human rights, including the integration of sexuality and sexual health into mental health education and services.

Psychiatrists should listen with compassion and humility and explore the needs of clients and their families. Carers may not always be listened to and they themselves frequently need time, information, education and continued support (Morrissey, 1997). Many people with enduring mental health problems lose their friends and social relationships (Jenkins, 1992) and many of these individuals are the most downtrodden within our society.

The roots of psychiatry can be traced back to the previous century. Within the traditionalistic 'law and order' climate of society and the sciences, human misery was medicalised into various mental illnesses. The sexual life of the mentally ill, if acknowledged at all, was regarded as dangerous or disturbed, a sign of decadence or an animal-like drive.

The possibility that the mentally ill might marry each other, generally, met with disapproval and opposition from family and healthcare workers. In his essay on 'Civilised sexual morality and modern nervousness', Freud (1908) stressed that 'we urgently advise our male patients not to marry any girl who has nervous trouble' (Vandereycken, 1993). Homosexuality in any form was considered a mental illness or deviant behaviour. As recently as 1978, an English psychiatrist went to court to prevent the marriage of two of his patients (Shanks and Atkins, 1985).

Despite the so-called sexual liberalisation in western societies and the revolutionary changes in mental health or psychiatric hospitals, the professional literature has given little attention to the sexual lives of people with mental health problems.

Drugs and sexuality

The introduction of psychotropic drugs in the fifties created a dramatic change in psychiatric hospitals. Clinicians quickly realised the negative effect of neuroleptics on the patients' sex life and began to use them for excessive or deviant sexual behaviour. Today psychotropic drugs are widely used, but how many people are informed about their effect on their sex life?

Compared to other side-effects, the importance of this issue has been underestimated or ignored. It is now clear that many drugs used in mental health can effect sexual functioning, for example anti-depressants (Gitlin, 1995), lithium in relation to men (Aizenberg et al, 1996), and medication contributed to sexual problems for 53% of clients diagnosed with schizophrenia (Buffum, 1993). Indeed, changes in sexual function may be a major reason why clients do not continue taking their medication. Research indicates that more male, than female clients with schizophrenia have sexual dysfunction associated with pharmacotherapy. The most common are erectile and ejaculatory problems (Lyketsos et al, 1983). However, it has been found that one third of females reported impaired sexual functioning during treatment with neuroleptics (Charirian et al, 1982).

Sexual side-effects are usually omitted from the promotional literature for physicians, unless the product has been proven 'harmless' in this respect. Although there have been more studies on these side-effects in recent years, systematic investigations are frequently restricted to sexual complaints in males. Similar bias can be found in research on physiological factors associated with sexual dysfunctions.

When a psychotropic drug is offered to a new patient, the advantages are stressed while vague and limited information may be given on its untoward effects. Sexual side-effects are commonly overlooked and may be difficult for the client or relative to cope with, possibly due to embarrassment.

There is a general lack of written information in relation to medication and other issues for clients and relatives in mental health services (Morrissey, 1997). More recently, the lack of literature concerning the attitudes and experiences of psychiatric staff with respect to sexual behaviour of hospitalised patients has been noted (Vandereycken 1993).

Research

In the UK and America, research indicates that people with long-term mental health problems are vulnerable to sexual exploitation (Kalichman et al, 1994), and many have poor knowledge about the transmission of sexually-transmitted diseases (STDs), including human immunodeficiency virus (HIV) (Cournos et al, 1994).

Furthermore, periods in hospital often make it difficult for people to have privacy, reducing opportunities to express love, affection or to be sexual. All forms of intimacy and social bonds can be adversely affected by admission to hospital. It is vital that health professionals recognise such effects on mental health.

To miss the company of a lover or friend is surely no mental disorder. Satisfactory sexual relationships contribute to mental and emotional well-being. There is a great need to address deficits within mental health services given that there is an absence of effective sexual health promotion in practice (Woolf and Jackson, 1996; Goisman et al, 1991; MIND, 1992). In particular, there is a need to develop sound and consistent management policies, professional training, sexual health promotion and an informed and proactive approach to mental health which integrates a broad understanding of sexuality. It has been shown that there is a lack of consistent agency policy and management support (Department of Health, 1994), which may explain why some clinicians opt out of this area of work.

Mental health services have, and should assume, a responsibility where service users are as safe as possible from sexual harassment, sexual exploitation and sexual abuse (Royal College of Nursing, 1996). However, funding for mental health services, government policy and

Safety

Fear about safety is something to which we can all relate. However, when a person has a fear for their sexual safety, health professionals should take them seriously and not ridicule the person or make them feel guilty. Health professionals have a responsibility to protect service users from sexual harassment, exploitation or abuse, although nurses may not feel that they can remain watchful for 24-hours-a-day, given the multitude of demands made on their time. Safety is an issue for all staff and all service users.

Hospital is seen as a place of safety yet there is growing concern, and evidence, that individuals with mental health problems may be victims of abuse in these settings (Edwards and Fasal, 1992; McMullen, 1990). Furthermore, there are many ethical issues for mental health nurses in relation to sexuality and mental health (Batcup *et al*, 1994).

Women service users have been on the receiving end of sexually abusive behaviour from male service users and male nursing staff. These included unwanted sexual comments, jokes, touching and rape (UKCC, 1993; Edwards and Fascal, 1992; MIND, 1992).

It has been reported that women service users have been sexually harassed and raped on mixed wards and staff have not intervened (MIND, 1992). Reports of incidents of sexual harassment by male staff towards female nurses have increased (UKCC, 1993).

Clearly, some people may be increasingly vulnerable to sexual exploitation, for example individuals with learning disabilities (MIND, 1992). There is also a clear link between childhood sexual abuse and mental health problems, although this may frequently be underestimated by health professionals (Campling, 1992). As yet there are few research-based nursing articles on sexual abuse issues, which clearly articulate the nurse's role (Sharkey, 1997). There is little evidence that hospitals or mental health services have staff guidelines, extensive policies or training in relation to sexual harassment, and preventative strategies and interventions to stop sexual assault on staff and users of mental health services are inadequate (Department of Health, 1994; Royal College of Nursing, 1996).

Sexual health promotion in mental health

People with mental health problems often need encouragement, practical support and time from professionals, such as mental health nurses. This means building a therapeutic relationship that will empower people to make decisions, choices, be informed and change their behaviour to meet their needs.

For experienced mental health nurses there are many barriers to promoting sexual health. For some individuals, their need for attention, affection, love and security overrides their need for personal safety and the safety of others. It is vital to recognise that many individuals with enduring mental health problems, such as schizophrenia may also be impoverished financially, and often lack good social networks and effective day-to-day living skills (Newton, 1988; Jenkins, 1992).

Recently, it has been shown that service users in mental health with enduring mental health problems, such as schizophrenia, have poor knowledge concerning the transmission of STDs, including HIV (Cournos et al, 1994). This suggests that clients may be unaware of the degree of risk to which their own sexual behaviour may put them, and that health professionals are inadequately organised for providing sexual health information and education (Morrissey, 1997; Royal College of Nursing, 1996).

Unfortunately, mental health service users in many settings have restricted or zero access to local family planning or sexual health services. Staff may be unaware or operate a referral system. Contraception and safer sexual resources, such as condoms and lubricants are either absent or inaccessible to service users and many obstacles exist in trying to implement a sexual health programme in mental healthcare. However, recent efforts have had significant positive benefits.

Woolf and Jackson (1996) carried out and evaluated the implementation of a sexual health programme in an acute psychiatric setting in an inner city. Subjects covered in the programme were safer sex, knowledge of HIV/AIDS and other sexually-transmitted diseases, assertiveness and practical skills in the use of condoms. Contrary to many negative assumptions about clients with mental health problems, it was found that these individuals attended group sessions with enthusiasm and were able to participate in the programme. This study also showed that mental health nurses possessed the skills to offer sexual health advice.

Many mental health professionals recognise their potential role in sexual health promotion with clients, but are hindered by a lack of policy and practice guidelines on sexual health work, a lack of professional training on sexual health, sexuality and related issues, resistance from colleagues and/or managers and concerns about the possible harmful effects of promoting sexual relationships for service users. Sexual relationships between psychiatric patients is a controversial topic involving legal and ethical issues, such as pregnancy.

In 1983 the California Court of Appeals dealt with a case where a woman who became pregnant at the mental health facility sued the physicians for failing to provide adequate supervision.

The Court ruled that the hospital was not responsible for her pregnancy and that hospitals should not impinge on patients' personal rights. The Court also stated that mental health professionals are expected to opt for treatments and conditions of confinement which are least restrictive of patients' personal liberties, maximising an individual's autonomy and reproductive choice. But it was considered that it was the hospital's responsibility to provide contraceptive counselling (Binder, 1985). However, such a ruling fails to recognise the true effect of mental health problems, such as schizophrenia on an individual's ability to make informed choices. Clearly, the health professional has a moral and legal right to protect those who are most vulnerable. Frequently, relatives feel fearful for the safety of the client during acute episodes where the person may lose touch with reality.

Sadly, there exist only a few reports on how hospitals cope with sexual intimacy between psychiatric inpatients. In a Canadian study by Keitner and Grof (1981), the percentage of hospitals that separated patients was roughly the same as the percentage of units that supported relationships (about 20%). In the remaining 60%, respondents would not commit themselves to one particular method, preferring to leave as many options as possible open in dealing with individual situations.

In the absence of clear guidelines, pressures of the moment are most likely to dictate how situations are handled. In their unit, Keitner and Grof provide patients with a written policy which includes the following statement, 'If you develop a relationship with another patient, staff will get together with you to help you decide whether this relationship is beneficial or detrimental to you and whether it would be to your advantage to continue or discontinue the relationship.' However, this is difficult when the patient neither wants your approval or is willing to listen. Such problems are complex, as the following examples illustrate.

1. For Tom it is his sixth hospital admission for alcohol abuse. He is unemployed. On the ward he is often seen in the company of Ann, an alcoholic receiving compulsory treatment due to extreme neglect of her children. The staff suspects a relationship between Tom and Ann, but there is no concrete evidence with which to confront them.

    When Ann can no longer be detained in hospital, she leaves the hospital. Tom remains but visits Ann at the weekends. All critical questions and warnings from the staff are experienced as 'them grudging him a new chance in life.' For this reason he thinks about leaving the hospital, but hesitates.

One weekend he returns to the hospital drunk. He was drinking with Ann, when a small argument turned into a serious fight. The next day Ann is found in a coma and is admitted to another hospital.

2. Michelle is under treatment for anorexia nervosa. One day a nurse finds her playing naked in the shower with John. When the incident is discussed in the staff meeting, many different opinions emerge. For the psychologist it is a positive sign that Michelle can respond playfully with a body she formerly detested. But others think John has abused Michelle's naiveté as he has done with other girls. Since he has so often breached ward rules, the psychiatrist decides to dismiss him. In the following weeks Michelle draws back into herself and loses weight again.

Clearly, there are many more examples in practice which cause concern for health professionals. There are issues connected with sexually disinhibited behaviour, masturbation, exhibitionism, inappropriate touching and sexually abusive language to staff and other clients.

Nurses can intervene to assist many of these clients to recognise and manage their sexual impulses in a socially acceptable manner. Sometimes antisocial sexual behaviour is a way of expressing sexual needs and a way to get attention, caring and love. In general, there is a lack of knowledge in relation to the sex lives of psychiatric patients. Sexual needs or desires are considered unimportant.

It is presumed that patients' sex lives are problematic or disturbed and should be viewed or treated as a secondary phenomenon, ie. a symptom or a consequence of the mental disorder. In the case of hospitalised psychiatric patients, difficulties in experiencing or expressing sexuality may, indeed, be due to the problematic situation for which they have been admitted. But often, it is an adaptive reaction to a major life change. If many patients in a psychiatric hospital can apparently live with little or no possibilities of sexual expression, it should be viewed as symptomatic of their institutionalisation (Vandereycken, 1993).

Furthermore, being a patient means having to live to certain rules, many of which prevent the maintenance of close relationships or severely restrict the patient's privacy. However, the sexual life of many patients is still surprisingly 'healthy' considering the personal problems and complicated living situations with which they have to contend (Ernst, 1988). It is, however, unclear what is meant here by healthy.

It is important to examine ways to assess the sexual health needs of people with mental health problems. In the following example, the assessment is for clients with schizophrenia. Such an approach could be adapted for clients with depression or other types of mental health problems. Perceptions and beliefs often colour objectivity (Jacobs, 1991) and mental health nurses should examine their attitudes towards their own sexuality and that of their clients. Sexual health needs to be incorporated into the nursing assessment process. A brief sexual history may be more appropriate depending on the situation, resources and the mental health of the client. The sexual history can include identification of the clients' physical, emotional, intellectual, social and spiritual needs (Beck *et al*, 1988). Following the assessment, mental health nurses need to identify a nursing diagnosis, client-centred goals and, based on this, develop a care plan. It is important to promote communications about sex and sexuality, correcting myths and misinformation within a confidential therapeutic relationship. Both the nurse and the client can evaluate the effectiveness of the sexual healthcare provided, which can include the input of a psychologist or sex therapist, depending on the problem.

Sex therapists believe that sexual research should focus more on areas, such as sex education (Apt Hulbert and Clarke, 1994). However, for mental health nurses, there is a real demand for assessment of sexual relationships and issues surrounding sexuality. In practice, this is handicapped by the lack of research studies on the sexual lives of people with mental health problems. An important first step is the assessment of an individual's sexual health needs. The example used here is an assessment for clients with schizophrenia, which is often overlooked. The assessment sheet is adapted from Beck *et al* (1988).

Assessing sexual health needs of clients with schizophrenia

Dimensions	Information needed
Physical	Previous baseline level of functioning Problems interfering with sexual functioning Use of illicit drugs and alcohol Effects of medication Body image
Emotional	Meanings associated with sexual acts Feelings about sexual activity Fears about sex acts and their consequences Effects of previous therapy

Dimensions	Information needed
Intellectual	Knowledge abouts STDs, HIV/AIDS Knowledge about contraception, pregnancy and parenting Understanding about safer sex Knowledge of ways of getting advice and help
Psychological	Quality, stability and type of relationships
Social	Cultural background Social skills, ability to form trust Rape or sexual abuse experiences
Spiritual	Beliefs, values, ritual traditions

Contrary to some professionals' beliefs, people who develop mental health problems, such as schizophrenia, tend to retain their sexual drive and its particular heterosexual or homosexual direction (Jacobs, 1991). When the wide range of schizophrenic states are considered, it appears that most individuals who have schizophrenia are not so different from other people in terms of their heterosexual or homosexual behaviour (Skopec et al, 1976). One difference is that some individuals can become preoccupied with sex in highly distorted and bizarre ways. Although many of their preoccupations and delusions appear to centre around sexual acts and pregnancy, there seems to be little propensity to act out these interests.

Many individuals diagnosed with schizophrenia prefer caring and comfort rather that overt sexual activity, with much of their sexual activity expressed in fantasy or masturbation. Research indicates that males with schizophrenia engage in autoerotic sexual activity two or three times as frequently as men in the general population (Lukianowicz, 1963). Clients with schizophrenia report that masturbation is not so much pleasurable as necessary (Skopec et al, 1976), and some clients indicated that masturbation counteracted the extrapyramidal side-effects of psychotropic drugs (Verhulst and Schneidman, 1981).

Sexual self-gratification may also result from the lack of opportunity for heterosexual or homosexual contacts, and from a difficulty in developing or maintaining intimate relationships with other people in their environment. An important area to discuss in relation to sexuality is that of the sexual boundaries for clients and health professionals.

Sexual boundaries

Boundaries are a real issue in the area of sex and sexuality given that the hospital setting encourages intimate relationships, while at the same time it expects these not to become eroticised or sexually expressed. Both staff and patients are caught in a catch-22 situation, where the therapeutic conditions promote intimacy while the rules dictate distance. Although sexualised therapist-patient relationships have become the focus of increasing concern, few reports consider staff-patient sexual interactions in patient units (Averill *et al*, 1989; Munsat and Riordan, 1990). Lack of clear boundaries can lead to aggression among staff and patients (Hummelen and Tietema, 1992).

Some guidelines have been put forward to assist clinicians and counsellors (Gray and House, 1991). More recently, in a legal context, there has been a need to acknowledge the sexual boundaries between mental health professionals and their involvement in sexual relationships with their patients. Strategies need to be considered in dealing with boundary violations (Gutheil and Weisstub, 1996). Mental health nurses are also aware that there are many types of issues which present difficulties for staff and other clients, and one of these is the issue of sexual abuse and sexual offenders (Rich, 1994). Specialist knowledge, skill and experience is needed in caring for many of these clients and there is an obvious need for, not only specialist services and education, but also a recognition of the need for training and resources for staff.

Human sexuality is multifaceted. A lack of social and interpersonal skills can severely hamper clients, preventing them from developing friendships and close intimate relationships. This can lead to loneliness, low self-esteem and depression. The mental health nurse, if available, can help clients to establish and maintain interpersonal peer relationships. It is distressing for carers, such as parents to watch their son or daughter lose their identity, friends and, all too often, their partner as a result of the effect of schizophrenia. Sadly, some clients with mental health problems may be unaware and insensitive to the needs of others because they are often unable to imagine themselves in someone else's place. Role play is a useful way to help these clients to develop interpersonal skills.

Basic material for role playing may include: how to approach an unknown person; how to respond when approached by an unknown person; how to verbalise interest, or lack of interest in another person, and how to make needs and desires known to another person. The role of sex education and training is important in mental health and can be either informal, when a client asks a direct question, or a programme set up to target specific issues, such as safer sex. HIV/AIDS prevention, information about STDs and group work, which could include workshops on relationships for users and staff, would all improve the quality of life for those suffering from mental health problems. Surely it is time for health professionals to recognise, encourage and respect all relationships, including sexual relationships in mental health.

References

Apt Hulbert DF, Clarke KI (1994) Neglected subjects in sex research: A survey of sexologists. *J Sex Marital Ther* **20**(3): 237–43

Averill SC, Beale D, Benfer B *et al* (1989) Preventing staff-patient relationships. *Bull Menninger Clin* **53**: 384–93

Aizenberg D, Sigler M, Zemishlany Z, Weizman A (1996) Lithium and male sexual function in affective patients. *Clin Neuropharmacol* **19**(6): 515–9

Batcup D, Thomas B (1994) Mixing the genders, an ethical dilemma: How nursing theory has dealt with sexuality and gender. *Nurs Ethics* **1**(1): 43–52

Beck C, Rawlins R, Williams S (1988) *Mental Health-Psychiatric Nursing: A Holistic Life-Cycle Approach*. Mosby, St. Louis:

Binder RL (1985) Sex between psychiatric inpatients. *Psychiatr Q* **57**: 121–6

Buffum MD (1993) Commentary on self-reported sexual behaviours of schizophrenic clients and non-institutionalised adults. *Wom Health Nurs Scan* **7**(6): 18

Campling P (1992) Working with adult survivors of child sexual abuse. *Br Med J* **149**: 886–9

Carmen F, Brady SM (1990) AIDS risk and prevention for the chronically mentally ill. *Hosp Comm Psychiatry* **41**(6): 652–7

Cournos F, Guido JR, Coomaraswamy S *et al* (1994) Sexual acts and risk of HIV infection among patients with schizophrenia. *Am J Psychiatry* **151**(2): 228–32

Charirian A, Chouinard G, Annable L (1982) Sexual dysfunction and plasma prolactin levels in neuroleptic-treated schizophrenic outpatients. *J Nerv Ment Dis* **170**(8): 463–7

Department of Health (1992) *The Health of the Nation*. HMSO, London

Department of Health (1994) *Working in Partnerships: Report of the Mental Health Nursing Review Team*. HMSO, London

Edwards M, Fasal J (1992) Keeping an intimate relationship professional. *Open Mind* **57**: 10–11

Ernst K (1988) Liebe in der psychiatrischen Klinik. In: Ernst K, ed. *Praktische Klinikpsychiatrie*. Springer-Verlag, Berlin:

Freud S (1908) *Civilized Sexual Morality and Modern Nervousness.* Vol 9, 179; 12(351): The Pelican Freud Library, Penguin, Harmondsworth

Gitlin MJ (1995) Effects of depression and antidepressants on sexual functioning. *Bull Menninger Clin* **59**(2): 232–48

Goisman RM, Kent A B, Montgomery EC *et al*, (1991) AIDS education for patients with chronic mental illness. *Comm Ment Health J* **27**(3): 189–97

Gray LA, House RM (1991) Counselling the sexually active client in the 1990s: A format for preparing mental health counsellors. Special Issue: Mental health counsellor training across the career lifespan. *J Ment Health Couns* **13**(2): 291–304

Gutheil TG, Weisstub DN (1996) Sexuality in the mental health system: patients and practitioners. *Int J Law Psychiatry* **19**(2): 183–90

Hummelen JW, Tietema W (1992) Sexuality and aggression among staff and patients. *Therapeut Comm Int J Therapeut Supp Org* **13**(1): 27–31

Jacobs P (1991) Sexual needs of the schizophrenic client. *Perspect Psychiatr Care* **27**(1): 15–20

Jenkins R (1992) Developments in the primary care of mental illness: a forward look. Int Rev Psychiatry 4(3/4): 237–42

Kalichman SC, Jeffrey KA, Johnson JR, Bulto M (1994) Factors associated with risk for HIV among chronic mentally ill adults. *Am J Psychiatry* **152**(2): 221–7

Keitner G, Grof P, (1981) Sexual and emotional intimacy between psychiatric inpatients: formulating a policy. *Hosp Comm Psychiatry* **32**: 188–93

Lukianowicz N (1963) Sexual drive and its gratification in schizophrenia. *Int J Soc Psychiatry* **9**: 250–58

Lyketsos G, Sakka P, Mailas A (1983) The sexual adjustment of chronic schizophrenics: A preliminary study. *Br J Psychiatry* 143: 376–82

McMullen HJ (1990) *Male Rape: Breaking the Silence of the last Taboo.* GMP, London

MIND (1992) *Stress on Women: Policy Paper on Women and Mental Health.* MIND Publication, London

Morrissey M (1997) A survey of information provision in mental health: What have we learned? *Int J Psychiatr Nurs Res* **3**(3): 361–9

Munsat EM, Riordan JJ (1990) Under wraps: prevalence of staff-patient sexual interactions on inpatient units. *J Psychosoc Nurs* **28**(9): 23–6

Newton J (1988) *Preventing Mental Illness.* Routledge, London

Royal College of Nursing (1996) *Sexual Health: Key Issues Within Mental Health Services.* RCN, London

Rich KD (1994) Outpatient group therapy with adult male sex offenders: clinical issues and concerns. Special Issue: Counselling men. *J Special Groupwork* **19**(2): 120–8

Shanks J, Atkins P (1985) Psychiatric patients who marry each other. *Psychol Med* **15**: 377–82

Sharkey VB (1997) Sexuality, sexual abuse. Omissions in admissions? *J Adv Nurs* **25**(5): 1025–32

Skopec H, Rosenberg S, Tucker G (1976) Sexual behaviour in schizophrenia. *Med Asp Hum Sex* **10**(1): 32–47

United Kingdom Central Council for Nursing, Midwifery and Health Visiting (1993) *Professional Conduct Occasional Report on Selected Cases*. UKCC, London

Vandereycken W (1993) Shrinking sexuality: The half-known sex life of psychiatric patients. *Therapeut Comm* **14**(3): 143–9

Verhulst J, Schneidman B (1981) Schizophrenia and sexual functioning. *Hosp Comm Psychiatry* **32**: 259–62

Woolfe L, Jackson B (1996) Coffee and condoms: the implementation of a sexual health programme in acute psychiatry in an inner city area. *J Adv Nurs* **23**: 299–304

Part 3
Evaluating practice

10
Sexuality, nursing and professional practice

Shirley Crouch

Introduction

The subject of sexuality and the individual has largely been marginalised by nursing. This chapter stresses the importance of nurses acknowledging the importance of sexuality in theory and practice. To deny it, is detrimental to the holistic care nurses should aim to provide. Sexuality is a topic high on the media agenda. Sex is used as a tool to bring down governments, sell toiletries, promote insurance products and highlight the immorality of society in general.

Sexuality is powerful, but it can also be powerless and impoverished, particularly if it belongs to a disadvantaged individual. Sexual media coverage can highlight the importance of youth and denigrate the aged or infirm. Although it can highlight the plight of the abused child, adolescent, youth, elderly and mentally impaired, it can also feed the needs of the perverse within society. If we accept that society has a powerful influence on an individual's sexual actualisation, nurses must also recognise the importance of the role that they play in assisting the individual in society to meet sexual actualisation. The average nurse may already be struggling with his/her own changing sexual role needs, but is in a position to discover or be asked about problems of sexuality from those in his or her care.

It is, therefore, paramount for the nurse to feel at ease in handling such issues, and to do this he/she must be able to identify his/her own self-belief and value systems with respect to sexuality. In this way, a truly humanistic approach to care will evolve. Discovery develops confidence and, as confidence grows, so does the ability to recognise one's own limitations and acknowledge the skills and knowledge of other professionals. All professionals should work together to prevent marginalisation of sexuality needs through a lack of awareness, embarrassment or the inability to feel at ease with discussing sexual issues.

Patients/clients can be vulnerable to the power of healthcare professionals who have not looked at their own assumptions, beliefs and value systems. Nurses have a professional responsibility to meet the sexuality needs of those in their care. The United Kingdom Central

Council for Nursing, Midwifery and Health Visiting Code of Conduct clearly states this responsibility.

> *Act always in such a manner as to promote and safeguard the interests and well-being of patients and clients; Tenet[1]*
>
> *Recognise and respect the uniqueness and dignity of each patient and client, and respond to their need for care, irrespective of their ethnic origin, religious beliefs, personal attributes, the nature of their health problems or any other factor; Tenet[7]*
>
> UKCC (1992)

Hazel Eaton (cited in Lucas, 1996) clearly feels asexual. Here the nurse's disregard of Hazel's dignity and individuality, and the removal of self is evident. It is important for nurses to take action on the Code's guidance and truly treat the individual as an individual and not an operation, medical disease or a task .

Just another resident

> *Two nurses link my arms, and with practised jerk and twist*
> *I am seated on the lavatory, dignity stripped*
> *They talk amongst themselves*
> *I am no longer the woman who bore four children*
> *The woman who had the strength to bring up a family on ration books*
> *Or the young woman who enticed men and turned heads*
> *Nor the woman in mature years, that wrote poetry and prose*
> *I, who was praised for her command of the English language.*
> *I sit here like a child seated on a potty looking up at you*
> *Begging you to notice me*
> *My mind works tho instead of words,*
> *My lips open and make strange sounds*
> *... I want to talk with you ...*
> *Ah good girl all done and again I am seated back in the chair*
> *These are last words spoken to me that night.*
>
> Hazel Eaton

Sexuality — towards a nursing definition

To understand human sexuality, nurses need to consider a range of biological, psychological and sociocultural factors. These factors may influence the nurse's own sexuality as well as that of the client.

To have a healthy or positively developed sense of sexuality has many benefits to the individual. Ingram-Fogel (1990) identifies them as follows:

- enabling a link with the future through children
- a means of physical release and sexual pleasure
- togetherness
- the communication of intense subtle feelings
- a feeling of self-worth when sexual experiences are positive
- the development of self, the individual identity we all have

Sexuality may mean different things to different people within different cultures and societies. Sexuality is being human and part of our multifaceted makeup. Sexuality may reflect, not only our individuality, but also our level of cohesion to the value systems, beliefs and norms of society.

There are many definitions offered in the literature, some writers emphasising the importance of an individual's sexuality to his or her identity and how these components of a person cannot be separated. Stuart and Sundeen (1974) explain that:

> *Sexuality is an integral part of the whole person. Human beings are sexual in every way all the time. To a large extent, human sexuality determines who we are. It is an integral factor in the uniqueness of every person. The total characteristics of an individual — social, personality, and emotional — that are manifest in his or her relationships with others and that reflect his or her gender — genital orientation.*
>
> (Shope, 1975)

Shope, however, includes the importance of relationships with others. As Webb and Askam (1987) state, love between different people depends upon the integration of somatic, emotional, intellectual and social components comprising the sexuality of each individual. It is important when explaining sexuality, emphasis is not put upon the sex act. Hogan (1980) suggests that sexuality is:

> *much more than the sex act ... (It is) the quality of the human, all that we are as men and women encompassing the most intimate feelings to find meaningful relationships.*

Other writers acknowledge that there is a difference between gender identity and sex, and how we change our way of expressing sexuality throughout our life cycle. All aspects of the human being that relate to being boy or girl, woman or man is subject to lifelong dynamic change. Sexuality reflects our human character, not just the genital nature.

Sexuality and the well-being of the individual

A growing body of knowledge accepts that sexuality is very important for the well-being of the individual and his/her quality of life. Mace et al (1974) gives the following definition of sexual health:

Sexual health is the integration of the somatic, emotional, intellectual and social aspects of sexual well-being in ways that are positively enriching and that enhance personality, communication and well-being.

Fundamental to this concept is the right to sexual information and the right to pleasure (Mace et al, 1974). Mace et al believe that sexual health includes three basic elements:
1. A capacity to enjoy reproductive behaviour in accordance with a social and personal ethic.
2. Freedom from fear, shame, guilt, false beliefs and other psychological response which could impair sexual relationships.
3. Freedom from organic disorders, diseases and deficiencies that interfere with sexual and reproductive functions.

Sexual health, therefore, implies a positive approach to human sexuality and the purpose of sexual healthcare should be the enhancement of life and personal relationships, not merely counselling and care related to the reduction of sexually-transmitted diseases. Every individual is a sexual being and sexuality is an important dimension of each person's personality. Ingram-Fogel (1990) suggests that sexuality underpins much of who and what a person is and has significance throughout life. She recognises that a person's sexuality can bring great pleasure when it is expressed positively, but that it also has the potential to cause pain. Through our sexuality we express our most intimate feelings of individuality and the need for emotional closeness with other human beings. It involves a continual process of recognising, accepting and expressing ourselves as sexual beings.

Sexuality is not just about sexual intercourse or even about relationships between people. It is about our concept of ourselves as men and women, our masculinity or femininity, as we see ourselves or as we would like to be, our appearance and behaviour and the effect we hope we have in attracting those who matter to us. It is about the fears and fantasies we have about ourselves and others (Glover, 1985).

Different people hold different views on what constitutes the self. Just what it is, where it comes from and how it should be expressed are continually debated. Mead (1934) argued that self was composed of two component parts, one aspect of self was the product of our personality — a unique blend of traits, attitudes and orientations that distinguish us from everyone else. The other aspect was the social self — created and moulded by the processes of primary and secondary socialisation. Our notion of self-image probably stems from both these aspects of self. Generally, humans like to believe that our self-image is congruous with, and an expression of, our personality, but it is also accepted that our self-image is strongly affected by what others think of us. Self-image is then, our own assessment of our social worth.

Self-image is affected by whether or not others think we are worthwhile people. It is important for our confidence, our maturation and our sense of achievement (Price, 1990). Society acts as a mirror by which we judge ourselves. We care desperately what other people think of us. In a society that emphasises body presentation as a guide to social worth, we are forced to take our personal body image seriously. Failure to achieve a satisfactory image may affect our self-respect and with that, a number of life opportunities. An extract from the following poem has always had a great impact upon me. I hope the feelings explored within it have influenced my nursing practice. In respect of sexuality, it is clear that Kate's self-image is not seen as important by the nurses who care for her, consequently, a feeling of turmoil is created. She wants the nurses to see 'her'.

What do you see?

> *What do you see, nurses,*
> *What do you see?*
> *Are you thinking,*
> *When you are looking at me;*
> *A crabbit old woman,*
> *Not very wise,*
> *Uncertain of habit,*
> *With far away eyes,*
> *Who dribbles her food*
> *And makes no reply*
> *When you say in a loud voice*
> *I do wish you'd try ,*
> *Who seems not to notice*
> *The things that you do,*
> *And forever is losing*
> *A stocking or shoe,*
> *Who, unresisting or not,*
> *Lets you do as you will,*
> *With bathing and feeding,*
> *The long day to fill.*
> *Is that what you're thinking,*
> *Is that what you see?*
> *Then open your eyes, nurse,*

You're not looking at me.
As I'll tell you who I am,
As I sit here so still,
As I rise at your bidding,
As I eat at your will.
I'm a small child of ten
With a mother and father,
Brothers and sisters,
Who love one another.
A young girl of sixteen,
With wings on her feet,
Dreaming that soon now
A lover she'll meet.
Dark days are upon me,
My husband is dead,
I look at the future,
I shudder with dread,
For my young are all busy,
Rearing young of their own,
And I think of the years
And the love I have known.
I'm an old woman now,
And nature is cruel.
'Tis her jest to make old age
To look like a fool.
The body is crumbled,
Grace and vigour depart.
There is now a stone
Where I once had a heart.
But inside this old carcass,
A young girl still dwells,
And now and again
My battered heart swells.
I remember the joys,
I remember the pain,
And I'm loving and living
Life over again.
I think of the years,
All too few
Gone too fast,
And accept the stark fact
That nothing can last.
So open your eyes, nurses,
Open and see,

Not a crabbit old woman,
Look closer . . . see ME.

Kate, the writer of this poem, was unable to speak, but was occasionally seen to write. After her death, her locker at Napsbury Hospital, near St. Albans, Herts was emptied and this poem was found. (Published in *The Health Service Journal*, 18/25 December 1986).

Here then we can see how self-image is inextricably linked with sexuality and the effects society can have on the individual in formulating a healthy sexuality. Both poems illustrate how an individual feels when self, personality and sexuality is eroded, creating a withdrawal into one's self, a feeling of worthlessness and great sadness. Nurses do have a responsibility to enable an individual to have the right to self-expression. Price (1990) identifies three components necessary for forming and maintaining a normal/healthy body image. These are:

1. Body reality — the way in which our body is constructed, namely the way it really is. This affected by both nature and nurture factors.

2. Body ideal — how we think we should look. We hold a personal body ideal which may also affect how we think other people should look. Body ideal is constantly changing and susceptible to a variety of influences.

3. Body presentation — how we present our body appearance (dress, pose, action) to the social world. We are able to control body presentation within certain limits, and to reflect actively on how body presentation was received by others.

If nurses accept the normal body image components proposed by Price (1990) then he/she has a professional responsibility to assist the patient or client to maintain positive self-worth. This is particularly important when patients have undergone physical or psychological trauma to their self-image which effects either body reality, body ideal or body presentation. To do this, it is necessary for the nurse to examine her/his own sexuality beliefs and value systems.

Sexuality belief and value systems

As far as we know, every culture that has ever existed has policed the sexual behaviour of its members to a greater or lesser extent (Caplan, 1987), and every culture has developed its own, constantly shifting, concept of sexual normality. In certain western cultures, notions of naturalness are widely used to support what are, in fact, ethical or moral beliefs about the acceptability or otherwise of different sexual behaviours (Weeks, 1986).

As the construct of sexual normality shifts, so the institutional organisation of sexual behaviour changes within and across cultures and history. Shifting beliefs about sexuality are complicated by the historical process whereby the scientific paradigm achieved its current dominance over the mystical/religious for understanding and interpreting life (Wilton, 1996).

Socially unacceptable sexual behaviours come to be seen as expressing inherent physical or psychological malfunction, rather than as representing sins which might be forgiven or temptation open to all. This notion is inadequate since it takes no account of the array of meanings attached to some sexual erotic behaviour, different sex erotic behaviour across cultures and different historical moments. Religious dogma, however, has not been entirely superseded by medical logic. We are left with a complex and confusing picture wherein the devout of many faiths continue to believe homosexuality is a sin and some sexual acts are wrong. Some nurses may have strong religious beliefs which are counter to clients' practices.

The sexual life of an individual is influenced by his or her background and accumulated life experiences. It is influenced by the values of the society in which he or she has been brought up. It is also influenced by the attitudes of others and by the individuals own personality and views of life.

An individual's sexual life is uniquely personal to him or her and is a fundamental part of his or her makeup. It is a complex mix of the physical and the psychological which, in turn, are dependent on social upbringing. Childhood and family play a large part in influencing a person's sexuality. It is a mode of communication that has to be learnt as a person matures.

Although society has become more aware of sexual pleasures and practices and more information is available, there is still an inherent hypocrisy that pervades society today concerning sexual practices and sexuality. This is evident in as much as some subjects are taboo, some religions still ban contraception and homosexuality and some consider alternative partners for coitus abnormal.

Beliefs about sexuality will differ between individuals and individual cultures. Perceptions of what is right and what is wrong will depend upon the unique interactions between individuals and individual cultures. They will also depend upon the unique interactions between the individual, families, friends and the community, and will vary according to culture, socio-economic grouping and religious background. From this, we each develop our own value systems and these systems are used throughout life.

Atkinson *et al*, (1981) acknowledge that attitudes have emotional, motivational and intellectual aspects and they may, in part, be unconscious. Attitudes, preferences and prejudices affect all our social interactions.

Attitudes from our past

To appreciate the context of sexuality in today's society, it is necessary look at our history, particularly the history of the Victorian era. The Victorian era lasted from 1837 to early in the twentieth century. From both fiction and historical literature, we gain the impression that the Victorian era was a time of high moral codes of practice, where the sanctity of marriage and the family were considered to be the foundation of society, and were developed for the good of society. In reality, this concept was based on idealism, not on realism. Most marriages were made for social reasons, as a good, moral foundation on which society was built, rather than for strong religious reasons. The husband's was the principal role in the family network. Upon marriage, the woman gave up all rights to money and independence and was expected to fulfil her duties as a wife and mother. The Victorian era had double standards. Marriage was seen as the way to maintain morals. Women were expected to be virgins, sex before marriage was frowned upon and women who ignored these boundaries were labelled as whores. At this time, the age of consent was 12 years of age. It was not until the latter half of the nineteenth century that this was raised to 16 years of age.

Pearsall (1976) suggests that people were uninformed about the issues relating to sex, particularly less well-educated women. Doctors and clergy misinformed lay people with regard to contraception and sexual practices. By withholding knowledge, it was hoped that these people would remain ignorant of the facts, and not indulge in immorality. In this way a virtuous society could be cultivated based on scrupulous ethics. This created a society based on sexual hypocrisy. Victorian society was based on a framework of high ideals which relied on the conditioning of people to conform. Many of these values still remain, particularly in the elderly of today and some of their beliefs and values have been passed on to their children. Nurses are individuals and, like their clients, have absorbed the beliefs and values that have been passed on to them.

The nurse's attitudes, beliefs and value systems

If a nurse is to become non-judgmental, she/he must learn to recognise and acknowledge his/her own feelings and attitudes towards other people's life situations, beliefs and feelings of independence. It is necessary for a person to accept his/her own judgmental feelings before finding it possible to uncover the origins of such feelings. The nurse needs to clarify her/his own customs, values and beliefs and ask questions, such as, Why do I act in the way that I do? How did I come to adopt these patterns of thoughts and behaviours? Such clarification will enable the nurse to appreciate that a patient/client is also an individual who has developed attitudes and beliefs, some of which may be similar to the nurse's own, some of which may be different.

Values modify behaviour through a process of self-monitoring. Personal value systems allow or disallow certain actions. As with customs, values vary from culture to culture, group to group and person to person. It cannot be assumed that all people's value systems are the same as one's own and nurses need to respect the values of other people. Through clearly identifying our own values, we are better equipped to make decisions about how we live our lives. We are also better equipped to appreciate the difference between our value systems and those of other people.

Identifying our own belief and value systems is not enough, we must also try to appreciate the affects that these might have on others. The way we speak and act often reflects our own belief and values, and we should self-monitor our communications and actions in order to prevent causing harm to others in our care, for example, our views on sexuality and what we perceive as healthy. We may view certain lifestyles as unacceptable. A nurse is on difficult ground if she/he condemns others for their values, but to communicate her/his abhorrence is against The Code of Conduct (UKCC 1992) and is not, therefore, within the concept of caring for others.

Nurses should be non-judgmental. The United Kingdom Central Council for Nurses Code of Conduct (1992) clearly states in tenet[7] that 'nurses should recognise and respect the uniqueness and dignity of each patient and client, and respond to their need for care, irrespective of their ethnic origin, religious beliefs, personal attributes, the nature of their health problems or any other factor.' Also tenet[1] which states: 'act always in such a manner as to promote and safeguard the interests and well-being of patients and clients.' The Code does not specifically mention sexuality, but encompasses the basic human rights of the individual and reflects the views of the World Health Organization (1975) regarding human rights and sexuality. These include:

- basic information about biological and psychological aspects of sexual development, human reproduction, the variety of sexual behaviour, sexual dysfunction and disease
- positive attitudes towards sexuality, and the possibility for objective discussion of sexual matters
- personnel who show understanding and objectivity towards the expression of sexual complaints to inform and advise regarding sexuality and sexual problems
  - training for health service personnel in this field
  - sufficient knowledge and resources to deal with complex problems of sexuality.

(WHO, 1975)

However, these recommendations were made in 1975 and little has changed. One could argue that perhaps the WHO have not been persistent enough in ensuring that these guidelines were implemented. We still appear to live in a society that is narrow-minded and prejudiced with regard to sexuality.

Irwin (1992) has produced guidelines for practitioners for re-evaluating attitudes towards homosexual and lesbian clients. These guidelines could equally be applied to the attitudes of all individuals when re-evaluating their personal views of sexuality. Homosexuals and lesbians have specific needs, but so, too, do others in society; the physically disabled, the sensory impaired and those with a learning difficulty or psychological impairment.

Guidelines for re-evaluating attitudes to sexuality

1. Assess your own value systems to determine what you think and feel about sexuality.
2. Examine your own perceptions of lesbians, gay men, children, adolescents, the middle-aged and the elderly. Determine where these attitudes and preconceptions have come from, what purpose they serve and whether they concur with reality.
3. Respond to any sexist or homophobic remarks made in the care environment and point out that such remarks are not acceptable.
4. Abandon the presumption of heterosexuality (Savage, 1987), ie. assuming that all patients are heterosexual unless they conform to cliché images and stereotypes of gay people.
5. Evaluate the care guides in your clinical areas to patients:
   - has the patient's privacy and right to confidentiality been respected?

- have any of the patient's physical, psychological or social needs been neglected or gone unmet because of negative attitudes of healthcare workers to sexuality?
- have all homosexual, elderly patients' loved ones been extended the same information as their heterosexual counterparts?

6. Read widely — forget most of the information given in medical and nursing textbooks about gay people, children, adolescents, middle-aged and the elderly regarding sexuality, as this may be distorted.
7. Monitor the sources of sexism and homophobics in society, be prepared to challenge fear and ignorance when and wherever it is encountered.

Adapted from Irwin (1992)

This guidance, if used effectively can ensure that patients/clients' rights are not prejudiced by the nurse's lack of awareness of an individual's sexuality needs.

Patient's rights

Patient's rights and the importance of providing a high standard of individualised and holistic care are given great importance in the nursing literature, but the reality is somewhat different. Too often there is only a superficial lip service to acceptance of others as individuals with freedom to choose how they live and the manner of their relationships (Faugier and Wright, 1990).

Sexuality has been described as an uninvited guest in the nurse/patient relationship (Savage, 1989) and research has shown that nurses' attitudes towards sexuality are often conservative and inflexible (Webb and Askham, 1987). This is hardly surprising given that the area of sexuality is still considered taboo in our supposedly enlightened society. Healthcare providers, as members of society, often ignore sexuality and treat it as taboo. They make excuses, such as 'the patient never brought it up.' There is often a hidden agenda behind such a comment, possibly the nurse's inability to come to terms with discussing sex. No matter what the reasons are, we need to recognise our own attitudes and values so that the barriers which prevent patients/clients receiving holistic care can be broken down.

Because of negative outcomes of the media coverage of sexuality, attitudes and behaviours are slow to change. Many aspects of sexuality remain undercover and are seen as evil and abnormal. As a result, the unique pleasure sexuality can give to a partnership is often marred because partners are unable to express publicly to a healthcare worker those activities which are part of their lifestyle for fear of condemnation or ridicule. Much still has to be done to educate the public regarding sexuality and acceptable sexual practices.

It may well be that some patients do not really care what the nurses think of them or their chosen lifestyle, but as Faugier and Wright (1990) state: 'all patients have the right to anticipate respect and regard from those entrusted with their care'. Admission to hospital is generally accepted as being an extremely anxiety-provoking experience and this is likely to be heightened by the added stress of contending with prejudices and disapproving attitudes from hospital staff.

The feelings of vulnerability, isolation and loss of control, often associated with admission to hospital, may be more pronounced for gay patients, transvestites and those who may participate in sexual activities not deemed as 'normal' by some. Expressions of affection and caring, such as kissing or close physical contact may be discouraged implicitly or more directly by healthcare professionals.

Ill-health evokes great emotions within a caring, loving relationship. Often the only way to express caring or love is by intimate contact and touch. It should be the nurse's responsibility to enable partners to achieve closeness. Hopefully my partner will be able to lay next to me in bed and hold me close as I die as he has always done in life when I have been unwell or upset. If on the other hand I am alone, I hope a carer will feel comfortable enough to comfort me and not see it as perverse and unacceptable.

In today's society, close contact with another individual can be very difficult. Where does professional care move to personal care. There is very little literature on sexual relationships between patient and nurse, but this could be because the majority of society would view a sexual relationship as physical and not necessarily appreciate its emotional and psychological aspects.

According to Beauchamp and Childress (1983), patients' rights are based on the moral principles of autonomy, beneficence, non-malevolence, veracity and justice in appropriate attitudes. Behaviour of nursing staff and other professionals can and do violate these rights. When it comes to meeting the sexual needs of clients, some nurses do not always act in a way that promotes and safeguards the well-being and interests of patients as required by The Code of Professional Conduct (UKCC, 1992). Cases of misconduct connected with inappropriate relationships with clients are heard by the UKCC.

The last decade has also seen the inappropriate examination of women and men under anaesthetic denigrated and not approved as an appropriate learning medium for medical staff. Satisfying expressions of sexuality should be seen as a right and not just a privilege. The World Health Organization (WHO, 1975) has outlined the fundamental rights of the individual, including the right to sexual health, which includes:

- a capacity to enjoy and control sexual and reproductive behaviour in accordance with a social and personal ethic
- freedom from fear, shame, guilt, false beliefs and other factors inhibiting sexual response and impairing sexual relationships
- freedom from organic disorders, diseases and deficiencies that interfere with sexual reproductive functions.

If expressing sexuality is viewed as a basic human right, then opportunities for privacy and freedom to mix with the opposite sex should be provided within healthcare settings. At the moment in many places, particularly in institutional settings, doors to side rooms are usually kept open and people are in multi-bedded bays or rooms. This lack of privacy, plus the absence of available, willing and desired partners are obstacles to sexual behaviour.

Meeting sexuality needs

If meeting the sexuality needs of individuals is part of the nurse's role, then nurses must develop ways of meeting those needs. The people providing care will have been brought up in different times with widely different morals, values and freedoms. They will have to listen and learn before they can appreciate the views of other people, which may conflict with their own. As generations age, they will have all witnessed the transitions in society's morals and values and, depending on their age, they will have been less influenced by them than younger generations. Sensitive education of carers on the sexual morality of different age groups may, perhaps, limit a potential clash of views.

The sexuality of those who care for people will reflect the society of their formative years. Today's carers may accept a more liberal attitude towards sexuality for themselves while considering others to have different principles to themselves, particularly if the others are elderly. Thus the views of the carer and the individual being cared for are likely to conflict. Today, there is still a strong sense of the family unit, where support and development of children in a stable environment is upheld. However, sexual freedom for women, homosexuals and lesbians is supported in law. There is a continual call for prostitution to be legalised, but society is fearful of this, preferring to ignore the role prostitutes play in a 'sexual' society. Sex with children is outlawed, but some members of society still abuse them, using the child's powerlessness to continue with the assault on his/her rights. In order for one person to be aware of another's sexuality, that person has to be aware of these social issues and recognise his or her own sexuality and sexual role in this society. This is fundamental for a person who is to become a skilled carer.

It must be incumbent upon health and social service professionals to acknowledge individual differences and allow for them when assessing and planning the care of individuals. The communication skills of the healthcare professional must be of a high order, not only in asking appropriate questions, but also when taking note of relevant cues for further exploration. Without a positive approach and factual knowledge, the individual may not be adequately assessed and thus may be inappropriately treated. This may have grave implications for care.

Problems are caused because people receive help from professionals who have been raised with different social conventions. Lack of insight, knowledge and skills prevent health professionals from helping clients to address their needs and this lack affects the abilities of the health professionals to identify their own changing sexual needs. Social constraints compound their lack of insight, making them reluctant to admit their ignorance.

The strength and power of stereotyping has to be recognised and taken on board if health professionals are to be adequately prepared to cover all aspects of caring for a person.

The legacy from Victorian times, compounded by negative stereotyping, a lack of awareness of their own sexuality on the part of health professionals and the perception of individuals that they do not need sexual advice, could mean that inappropriate help is given for sexual problems or issues. As people become less inhibited about examining their own sexuality, perhaps this will become less of a problem and they will begin to accept others for what they are. Labelling others and making value judgments in the name of religion or morality will become unacceptable. People should be treated as individuals, respected as people and their needs valued. When this is the accepted norm appropriate care will be given.

Sexuality and nursing care

Many research reports document the general inadequacy of health professionals' abilities when considering the sexuality of those in their care (Webb, 1985; Webb and Askam, 1987; Booth, 1990; Lowis and Bor, 1994).

Payne (1976), in a study of relationships, investigated nurses knowledge, attitudes and statements of nursing behaviour about sexuality and their degree of comfort with sexual situations. She measured this using a Professional Sexual Role Inventory and a sex knowledge and attitude test. The main hypothesis set by Payne was that: 'the more knowledge a nurse has of human sexuality, the more favourable will be his/her attitude towards it and the more comfortable she/he will be in professional situations that are conjoined with sexual situations'. This was supported and confirmed in numerous other situations. Knowledge, if utilised effectively, is a very powerful and malleable tool.

Among nurses, students were more knowledgeable and liberal in their attitudes than registered nurses. Surprisingly, family planning nurses, who might be expected to possess the appropriate knowledge and be more comfortable with their own attitudes when discussing sexuality, were less knowledgeable than students. This could be because they still carry with them a baggage of inherited beliefs and values of sexuality. We must also ask whether family planning nurses, whose role at this time was advice on contraception, appreciated the significance of 'sexuality' for the individual or were only aware of the issue when it related to coitus.

Lewis and Bor (1994) undertook a study to determine the relationship between knowledge of, and attitude towards, sexuality and nursing practice. They specified nursing practice in discussion of sexuality with the patient, but identified that factors other than those within the study influence nursing practice. They suggested that knowledge and attitude about sexuality are related, but that little has changed in either over the last 20 years. The implications of the study suggest the need for improvement in nurse education and sexuality at all stages of training.

Webb (1985) called for sexuality to be part of the nursing curriculum because, before nurses are able to help others, they must examine their own attitudes towards the subject. Its inclusion in the curriculum has only happened recently and even now it is defined and taught in narrow terms, with many vital areas overlooked (Weston, 1993; Brogan, 1996).

Values concerning sex develop over the years and it takes experience and the opportunity for open discussion to learn how to handle the subject sensitively. Brogan (1996) quotes Castledine (1981) who asks, 'Is there sex after death', meaning will nurses learn to discuss sexuality openly as they are now doing with death?

There is some social conditioning with respect to sexuality, and educational preparation will help to dismantle the traditional views, thus improving nursing care and encouraging personal development of nurses themselves. Before this can take place, the leaders need to gain insight into their own attitudes and beliefs (Webb, 1985; Webb and Askam, 1987).

Education and training

Education is the key to change (Jones, 1988), but as Platzer (1996) notes, nurse education too must rid itself of prejudice and intolerant attitudes before it is able to move forwards, although this is insufficient in itself. The whole ethos of nurse education needs to change from promulgating conformity and similarity of thinking (Burnard, 1993), to promoting individuality, autonomous thinking and critical self- and social awareness.

A greater knowledge and appreciation of social psychology, which aims to analyse and understand human social behaviour, might facilitate an awareness in nurses of their own attitudes, prejudices and preconceptions, how these come about and how they can influence the care and support extended to patients and colleagues. Nurse education should disabuse nurses of existing myths and stereotypes about sexuality, replacing them with a varied and positive image of sexuality and the individual. Very little is written in the UK regarding sexuality, particularly for those people at the end of the age spectrum or those with a disability. Roper, Logan and Tierney in 1980 classified expressing sexuality as an activity of daily living and each human being as a sexual being.

One year later, however, Booth (1990) notes that the same authors produced a model care plan for a 73-year-old man who has suffered a CVA when living at home with his wife. Under expressing sexuality we read: of nil relevance. Booth identifies that this activity of living seems to have vanished altogether by 1988 in another work by Roper. Like Booth, I find this disconcerting for several reasons. In 1980 the three eminent authors recognise each human being as a sexual being and prior to this much had been written on self-image, sexuality and health. Yet the dramatic loss of self that the gentleman suffering from a CVA in the 1981 study must have experienced is insignificant. This is extremely worrying as it suggests acceptance of marginalising or ignoring the issue. Nursing has accepted holism as a basis of care, but there are still areas of care that are neglected. Culture and sexuality are only two such areas and, if we believe that both are part of being human, much still needs to be done in educating all nurses about the importance of these areas for the individual. As Booth highlighted, attitudes to sexuality were changed by the stroke of a pen.

Summary

Sexuality is a complex subject; it is a personal subject taught with prejudice and taboo. But it is part of life itself and should be of paramount importance to us all. Enlightenment will create a more caring and supportive society thereby allowing the self-actualisation we are all entitled to. Once nurses accept that they are dealing with patients as whole people, rather than just nurturing their disease, dealing with sexuality will cease to be traumatic.

Clearly nurses have a responsibility to help meet an individual's sexuality needs, but they should recognise that, without support, they are unable to do so. Interdisciplinary co-operation is necessary as it is the author's view that no one profession can be an expert on sexuality. Nurses need to recognise their unique role within the care team. If nursing purports to have a humanistic approach to practice, the humanistic approach should be employed, thus reducing the possibility of marginalisation of sexuality by lack of knowledge and skills.

References

Andrews J (1988) Sexuality and the older person. In: Wright S, ed. *Nursing the Older Patient*. Harper and Row, London

Atkinson RL, Atkinson RC, Hilgard ER (1981) *Introduction to Psychology*. Harcourt Brace Jovanovich International, New York: Chapter 3

Beauchamp TL, Childress JF (1983) *Principles of Bio-medical Ethics*, 2nd edn. Oxford University Press, New York

Booth B (1990) Does it really matter at that age? *Nurs Times* **86**(3): 50–2

Brogan M (1996) The sexual needs of elderly people: addressing the issue. *Nurs Stand* **10**(24): 42–5

Burnard P, Chapman CM (1993) *Professional and Ethical Issues in Nursing*, 2nd edn. Scutari Press, Harrow

Caplan P (1987) *The Cultural Construction of Sexuality*. Routledge, London

Castledine G (1981) Is there sex after death? *Nurs Mirror* **152**(14): 12

Faugier J, Wright S (1990) Homophobia, stigma and AIDS — an issue for all healthcare workers. *Nurs Pract* **3**(2): 27–8

Glover J (1985) *Human Sexuality in Nursing Care*. Croom Helm, London

Heron J (1977) *Behavioural Analysis in Education and Training*. Human Potential Research Project. University of Surrey, Guildford

Hogan R (1980) Nursing and human sexuality. *Nurs Times* **29**: 1296–300

Ingram-Fogel (1990) *CI Sexual Health Promotion*. WB Saunders, Philadelphia

Irwin R (1992) Critical re-evaluation can overcome discrimination. Providing equal standards of care for homosexual patients. *Prof Nurse* April: 435–8

Jones H (1994) Mores and morals. *Nurs Times* **90**(47): 55–8

Jones R (1988) With respect to lesbians. *Nurs Times* **84**(4): 20, 48–9

Lewis S, Bor R (1994) Nurses' knowledge of and attitudes towards sexuality and relationship of these with nursing practice. *J Adv Nurs* **20**: 251–9

Lucas R (1996) *Tranquil Echoes*. Ron Lucas Publications, Peterborough: 27

Mace Dr, Braverman RHO, Burton T (1974) *Teaching Human Sexuality in Schools for Health Professions*. World Health Organisation, Geneva

Mead GH (1934) *Mind, Self and Society*. University of Chicago Press, Chicago

Payne T (1976) Sexuality of nurses: correlation of knowledge, attitude and behaviour. *Nurs Res* **25**(4): 286–92

Pearsall R (1976) *Public Purity, Private Shame*. Weidenfield and Nicholson, London

Platzer H (1993) Women's health and sexuality. *Nurs Stand* **4**(5): 33–5

Price B (1990) *Body Image: Nursing Concepts and Care*. Prentice Hall, London

Roper N, Logan WW, Tierney AJ (1980) *The Elements of Nursing*. Churchill Livingstone, Edinburgh

Roper N, Logan WW, Tierney AJ (1981) *Learning to Use the Process of Nursing*. Churchill Livingstone, Edinburgh

Roper N (1988) *Principles of Nursing in Process Context*. Churchill Livingstone, Edinburgh

Savage J (1987) *Nurses, Gender and Sexuality*. Heinemann, London

Savage J (1989) Sexuality: an uninvited guest. *Nurs Times* **85**(5): 25–8

Shope D (1975) *Interpersonal Sexuality*. WB Saunders, Philadelphia

Stuart G, Sundeen S (1979) *Principles and Practices of Psychiatric Nursing*. CV Mosby, St Louis, MO

United Kingdom Central Council for Nursing, Midwifery and Health Visiting (1992) *The Code of Conduct*. UKCC, London

Waterhouse J, Metcalfe M (1991) Attitudes towards nurses discussing sexual concerns with patients. *J Adv Nurs* **16**: 1048–54

Webb C (1985) Teaching sexuality in the curriculum. *Sen Nurse* **3**: 10–12

Webb C, Askham J (1987) Nurses' knowledge and attitudes about sexuality in healthcare, a review of the literature. *Nurse Educ Today* **7**: 75–86

Weeks J (1986) *Sexuality*. Routledge, London

Weston A (1993) Challenging assumptions. *Nurs Times* **89**(18): 26–9

What Do You See (1986) *The Health Services Journal*, 18/25th December.

Wilton T (1996) Caring for the lesbian client: homophobia and midwifery. *Br J Midwif* **4**(3): 126–31

World Health Organisation (1975) *Education and Treatment in Human Sexuality: The Training of Health Professionals*. Technical Report Series No 572. WHO, Geneva

11
Perspectives on sexual health promotion

Theodore H MacDonald

Sexual health promotion in the context of HIV/AIDS

Nowhere can health promotion principles of empowerment and autonomy be more sensitively applied than in the modern context of HIV/AIDS. The British government, in its 1992 Health of the Nation document, identified sexual health as an important health concern in the UK. Health promotion has moved away from a victim-blaming focus on HIV prevention to a more participatory attitude within sexual health promotion. In this chapter, the author will incorporate broader prevention activities, such as reproductive health and sexually-transmitted diseases, as well as HIV infection itself.

The chapter aims to consider sexuality inclusively and not focus only on reproductive health. This will allow a more detailed analysis of the social and behavioural aspects of sexual health promotion and not merely the costs and other consequences of medical interventions.

Special attention has been paid to HIV and AIDS only to illustrate some of the problems inherent in sexual health promotion, such as risk behaviour and the relationship between knowledge and beliefs. Such an assessment of the effectiveness of sexual health promotion, allows us to highlight the difficulties in measuring health behaviour change. First, it is important to lay the foundation to this discussion by defining the terms used and then to give an overview of models and approaches used in sexual health promotion.

Obviously, any work relating to the promotion of sexual health has to recognise the diversity of human sexual behaviour and differing views on sexuality and, finally, what constitutes sexual health promotion. Sexuality itself is hard to define, but it is certainly much more complex than is suggested by its purely biological function. 'Sexuality is more a question of identity and links closely to a person's sense of self' (Aggleton and Tyrer, 1994). Sexual expression varies enormously and we finally appreciate that there are no links between sex or gender or sexuality. It is from this starting point that sexual health promotion must begin.

Focus of the debate

We begin by considering what is meant by sexual health. The Terence Higgins Trust (cited by Aggleton and Tyrer, 1994) recognises that sexual health includes 'physical and emotional well-being, as well as the avoidance of sexually-transmitted diseases and unwanted pregnancies, with an overall focus on the practice of safer sex.' George (cited by Alcorn, 1996) writes 'sexual health describes the effects that sexuality can have upon health and that health can have upon sexuality.' The World Health Organization concluded in 1987 (cited by Aggleton and Tyrer, 1994) that 'due to the range of individual, cultural and social differences and the various patterns of lifestyle, social and gender roles, there can be no single definition of a sexually healthy individual.'

For reasons such as these, sexual health promotion has been defined in a variety of broad terms. Like health and illness themselves, definitions cannot be specific because the terms are subjective and relative. French and George (cited in Alcorn, 1996) view sexual health promotion 'as an umbrella term to describe any intervention which aims to: promote sexual well-being; prevent HIV, other STDs, unwanted pregnancies'. Likewise, Curtis (cited by Alcorn, 1996) writes: 'When one considers that HIV is only the most serious of a range of sexually transmissible agents including several viruses which are as yet incurable, and that even curable infections such as gonorrhoea, chlamydia and syphilis continue to take their toll of pain, infertility and human misery, it is apparent that the significance of sexual behaviour for public health extends well beyond the prevention of AIDS, and that purely treatment-orientated approaches hold no solution to the problem.'

There is now a definition for HIV/AIDS health promotion that the World Health Organization created to cover the activities required to contain the spread of HIV: 'as the culture-specific process, which seeks to influence positively, the relevant health practices of individuals and groups so as to prevent the transmission of HIV infection' (cited by Pye and Kapila, 1990).

Are preventive strategies empowering?

Only 15 years ago, HIV prevention strategies were built on the preventative and educational models, which were based on coercion and blame rather than on support and empowerment. The first media campaigns used imagery, such as tombstones and references to plague, to frighten people into acquiescence. This caused people to either over or under react. The lessons learned were that proposed behavioural changes have to be attractive and individuals must believe that they are personally at risk. Indeed, individuals must feel that they can both achieve behaviour change at an acceptable cost and that behaviour change will avoid HIV infection. Telling people the facts and then assuming that this will lead to automatic behaviour change has proven to be relatively ineffective in sexual health education.

Likewise, the early prevention strategies had faults. They were biased towards making people 'differentially' responsible for their behaviour by implying social disapproval of certain lifestyles and apportioned blame to certain groups in society. Instead of stopping the spread of HIV, policy makers and the media alike seemed determined to stop certain activities and preferences, such as homosexuality, promiscuity, prostitution, drug use and so on. To counter this type of approach, education about sexual health must involve far more than the provision of facts and information.

It is now recognised that self-empowerment and community-based initiatives constitute the most effective interventions (Aggleton and Moody, 1992; McEwan and Bhopal, 1991). The self-empowerment model is favoured because it extends the educational approach by giving individuals choice and power, and the collective approach is preferable because campaigns need to be seen to be at a grassroots level so that people have the choice about how best to realise their local population agendas and to target needs. It is argued by many that social change should ideally come from the bottom up, rather than the top down and that it succeeds through the involvement of the community, those threatened and concerned and those whose everyday life is affected (Tones, 1981; McEwan and Bhopal, 1991; Aggleton and Moody, 1992; Kickbusch, 1994). Aggleton and Tyrer (1994) take this further and argue that 'for education about sexual health to be most effective, it is important to attempt to develop and promote an awareness of wider issues, such as oppression, gender inequality, distribution of power and cultural expectations.'

Sexual health promotion can take place in a number of different settings, for example, in general practice, family planning services and in genito-urinary clinics (GU). In the UK, the number of cases seen in GU clinics has doubled over the past 15 years and now amounts to nearly 740 000 new cases a year (Adler, 1995). The reason for this is multifactorial. For example, the introduction of the pill and other non-protective barrier methods of contraception is a factor. However, Adler also argues that improved service provision and contact tracing may also be responsible for the increased numbers presenting to GU clinics, so it is difficult to make assumptions about numbers in real terms.

The aim of sexual health promotion in GU clinics is to 'offer prompt diagnosis and treatment, minimise the incidence of complications, trace and treat the infected partners of patients, and educate patients, the public and healthcare workers' (Adler, 1995). Early diagnosis and treatment for many sexually-transmitted diseases is not only cheap, but also effective in controlling the spread of such diseases. Methods of control are through epidemiological treatment, which can help to reduce the infection 'pool' in the community, raising awareness through education and protecting the health of individuals who are unaware that they may be infected by gonococcal, chlamydia or syphilis, through contact tracing. The prevention of costly long-term disability is of crucial importance. For example, most cases of pelvic inflam- matory disease are preventable.

Problems arise when a sexually-transmitted disease that is left untreated, leads to long-term damage and suffering in women. This, in turn, means long-term support and a drain on medical resources. Evidence suggests that early diagnosis and prevention is the only effective way to manage this difficult condition (Adler, 1995; Mann *et al*, 1996).

Community barriers to sexual health promotion

Numerous problems are associated with encouraging people to participate in the promotion of their sexual health. For example, there are practical problems such as access to services. Although there are 240 departments of GU medicine in the UK, there is still a tendency for these services to be located in dingy basements or down dark alleyways. Facilities should alleviate, not create, stigma and be readily accessible for self-referral (Adler, 1995; McHaffie, 1993). Other problems for people attending clinics are embarrassment, fear and confidentiality. 'Some departments are called after physicians, apostles or battles and others are termed 'special departments' or given a number or letter' (Adler, 1995). This can confuse and alienate people when accessing a clinic.

There are also particular problems in the provision of healthcare for women in that the services are split between primary care, the gynaecologist, GU services and family planning. Thus, without integrated facilities and collaboration between specialities, contacting and treating sexual partners can be problematic or inefficient (Mann *et al*, 1996). The law can also inhibit access to support/healthcare services. Legislation on the age of consent makes it even more difficult to reach and promote sexual health to underage women or young gay men, who may be particularly vulnerable to infection.

It is the issue of HIV/AIDS which, more than any other factor, has forced society to address the areas of sex and sexuality in all its forms. The Health of the Nation has described HIV and AIDS as 'the greatest new threat to public health this century' (Health of the Nation, 1991). In the government's White Paper (1992) on the Health of the Nation, one of the five key areas identified for change is sexual health because of the rapid spread of HIV/AIDS. The objectives were to reduce the incident of HIV infection and other STDs by strengthening monitoring and surveillance and by providing services for the effective diagnosis and treatment of these infections. The target was to reduce:

- the national incident of gonorrhoea by at least 20% by 1995
- the proportion of drug users who report needle sharing from a fifth in 1990 to no more than a tenth in 1997
- by at least half, the rate of conceptions amongst the under 16s by the year 2000

Whether this was achievable will be discussed later. First, it is important to consider some of the fundamental dilemmas associated with the issue of HIV/AIDS. As Weeks pointed out (cited by Scott and Freeman, 1995) 'what gives AIDS a particular power is its ability to represent a host of fears, anxieties and problems in our current, post-permissive society.' As Scott and Freeman (1995) argued, these risks and problems are managed in different 'social arenas'; namely, in public policy, by medicine and by individuals.

Public health is orientated to controlling disease in such a way as to permit surveillance of sources of infection. In the case of HIV, unlike other infectious diseases, 'the usefulness of surveillance as a method of evaluation effectiveness is seriously limited by the particularities of infection with HIV, such as the stigma attached, the long latency period, the dynamic of the epidemic and the absence of a vaccine or an effective treatment' (Friedrich *et al*, 1994). So the question arises 'Should authoritarian approaches be enforced to minimise the spread of disease?' For example, criminalisation of a West Midlands man accused of deliberately infecting four women with the virus was discussed by government ministers in 1992 (Guardian, 1992; cited by Scott and Freeman, 1995) or in the liberal approach of prevention by identifying the individual's behaviour and looking to change this through the provision of information, education, advice and support. A strategy put forward for the 1990s about the nation's health states that, 'Human behaviour does not reflect individual choices alone so much as the powerful influence of the social, economic and political environments that lie substantially beyond the control of the individuals who are affected by them.' This recognises that the state of the nation's public health cannot rest on the responsibility of individuals alone. There must also be government action; the two must interact and need to work hand in hand (Department of Health, 1992).

Medicalisation v health promotion

Modern medicine has had little impact on the spread of HIV as it has not been able to find a cure or vaccine and is unlikely to do so for some years to come (Scott and Freeman, 1995; Holland and Fullerton, 1995). Medicine can define areas of risk and prevention but cannot remove it. 'Even where effective therapies do exist, for example against syphilis and gonorrhoea, their spread cannot be successfully contained by medical therapies alone' (Holland and Fullerton, 1995). Understanding risk-taking behaviour and preventing the spread of these diseases has called into play many other factors, such as contact tracing and raising awareness.

'Since diseases that are prevented are necessarily unreported, the success of a preventative procedure is more difficult to demonstrate than that of a therapy' (Department of Health, 1992). It is difficult to prove that those who remain healthy have done so because of a preventative programme. It is also argued that prevention seems less efficient than treatment, because money is being directed towards a healthy population and the outcome is not necessarily tangible or immediate, unlike medication for someone who is sick. 'The focus of health education has shifted from disease process to personal behaviour, as evidenced by the dominance of 'lifestyle' in discussions of prevention' (Scott and Freeman, 1995). However, health promotion within the context of the health service is still dominated by the biomedical model which is criticised for being narrow and too medicalised (Scott, 1992).

Generally, health education messages have been designed to promote safer sex, the core elements of which are negotiation and condom use. 'Safer sex is premised on an awareness and acceptance of risk and, in turn, on the production of trust. In this context, trust may be understood as the solution to a specific problem of risk. In turn, this raises the question of the relationship between risk awareness and risk avoidance' (Scott and Freeman, 1995). Individuals have to assess their own risk as it is impossible to arbitrarily assume that high risks of HIV infection attach to certain individuals. Health promotion can assist in this dialogue, but negotiation in any relationship can never be complete or absolute because it is dependent on so many hidden factors. 'One of the reasons why it is so difficult to translate anxiety about HIV and AIDS into rational dialogue is precisely because it calls trust and intimacy, the insecure bases of fragile sexual identities, into question' (Scott and Freeman, 1995).

Trust, intimacy and personal autonomy

Trust may, therefore, be viewed as a solution to the prevention of the transmission of HIV infection within relationships, but the problems here are that for many young women, for example, 'the need to trust has its roots in romantic, feminine discourse and is likely to result in an understanding of love as prophylactic' (Scott and Freeman, 1995). Trust is seen not only in terms of trusting a partner, but in people's perception of risk. For example, 'it won't happen to me', 'I'm clean', 'I'm straight'. 'Trust is neither in a relationship nor in a rational process of risk assessment, but in cultural understandings of sexuality and in gendered sexual scripts' (Scott and Freeman, 1995).

Holland *et al* (1992) explains in her study of the negotiation of safer sex, that for young women this is problematic because of their subordinate role and this can contribute to unsafe sexual behaviour, regardless of the dangers. 'The understanding of sexual risk-taking by young women and the promotion of safer sex for young heterosexuals will depend on the extent to which we can make connections between the sexual pressures on young women, their resistance to these pressures and their personal empowerment in managing their own lives' (Holland *et al*, 1992). Promoting sexual health is, therefore, a complex dialogue between the health promoter and the client and the ability of both to put those health education messages into practice.

Central to much HIV prevention work is the dynamic of power, not only for women but for everyone. Aggleton describes this as 'the power that denies women the opportunity to participate fully in sexual decision-making; the power that limits the freedom of lesbians and gay men to express their sexuality openly and without fear of attack; the power that denies those who are physically or intellectually disabled the right to a fulfilling sex life; the power that denies young people access to the information they may need to protect themselves against unwanted pregnancy and STD and the power that encourages an understanding of black people's sexuality as being different from and not inferior to that of whites.' It is important to understand these underlying issues when discussing sexual health promotion because any assessment of its effectiveness would have to recognise relative levels of empowerment (or its reverse) in the context of marginalisation of various types.

Perception of risk

Fundamental to the logic underlying the hypothesis of health promotion is the expectation that it alters people's perception of risk. 'Successful HIV intervention campaigns would need to address the situations in which risk behaviour occurs and, not least, the power relations which limit or eliminate health choices' (Bloor, 1995). The psychological context assumes immense importance.

For example, when individuals are faced with dealing directly with a problem they often go into 'denial —the problem does not exist, displacement — the problem has nothing to do with me and delay — I'll change my behaviour one day, but not right now' (Aggleton and Tyrer, 1994). There are many theories that are put forward to explain the variations in perceptions of risk. The Health Belief Model is most widely used to describe HIV-related risk behaviour (Bloor, 1995). For example, the Health Belief Model views health behaviour in association with interlinked perceptions.

'Firstly, the individual must perceive him/herself as vulnerable or susceptible to a health threat, such as HIV infection. Secondly, that health threat has to be perceived as having serious consequences. Thirdly, the protective action that is potentially available to avoid that health threat has to be perceived as an effective safeguard. And fourthly, taking the protective action has to be perceived to have benefits which outweigh the perceived costs' (Bloor, 1995). However, issues which must be considered are power dynamics within a relationship, for example, the negotiation of safer sex, constraint versus choice, immediate incentives of risk taking, etc. The immediate pleasure of sharing needles, for example, may outweigh any thought of the long-term risk.

Some would argue that the Health Belief Model does not work because 'there is inconsistent evidence that knowledge of risk is related to behaviour change' (Cohen and Chwalow, 1995). It is all too obvious that individuals often have a poor ability to perceive risk because people find it hard to recognise their own susceptibility. It could be said that health behaviour is the wrong domain and that many people have more immediate needs that outweigh the outcome of unprotected sex and they may be prepared to take risks accordingly. Knowledge, attitudes and beliefs are as much a consequence of behaviour as the cause of behaviour, basically they all measure the same thing. Information can result in dramatically different behaviours given different environments or times. Information is not static and a focus on the individual neglects the dynamics of social interactions that shape behaviour, as pressure from others can shape behaviour. With all this in mind, the question now remains, Does sexual health promotion work? Given the complexities and dynamics briefly outlined above, it is hard to prove, as shall now be explained.

The problem of assessment

There are a variety of processes by which the quality of HIV/AIDS health education and health promotion programmes are assessed. It is necessary to briefly explain the difference between monitoring and evaluation and to explain some of the key issues and techniques that are commonly used.

The World Health Organization has defined monitoring as: 'the process of collecting and analysing information about the implementation of the programme; it involves regular checking to see whether programme activities are being carried out as planned so that problems can be discerned and dealt with' (World Health Organization, 1986).

Evaluation is described as: 'the process of collecting and analysing information about the effectiveness and impact of either particular phases of the programme or the programme as a whole. Evaluation also involves assessing programme achievements for the purpose of detecting and solving problems and planning for the future' (World Health Organization, 1986).

Monitoring, therefore, is concerned more closely with the ongoing implementation of a programme, whereas evaluation is concerned with the programme's effectiveness. There are two types of evaluation frequently used in HIV/AIDS health education programmes — outcome and process evaluation.

There are many components to outcome evaluation but its principle aim is to measure changes that are cognitive, eg. knowledge about HIV and its modes of transmission; attitudinal, eg. views about people with HIV/AIDS; and behavioural, eg. changes in person or group behaviour (Aggleton and Moody, 1992). Alternatively, the outcome measure can be to estimate the number of people reached by a particular initiative or the amount of resources used (Aggleton and Moody, 1992). In all cases goals (statements of intent), objectives (desired end result) and performance targets (intermediate results) must be made so reliable and valid that indicators (data on changes that have taken place) can be achieved.

Process evaluation examines how and why the outcomes in the latter were achieved. It is more qualitative and descriptive rather than quantifiable. 'The emphasis in process evaluation, therefore, is on studying the process of learning that takes place through health education and health promotion and on identifying factors that facilitate or impede individual and group behaviour change' (Aggleton and Moody, 1992). It looks at the 'how' and 'why' questions, that is, it explores different perspectives of the empowerment and community action approaches and incorporates the overall picture of management, workers as well as clients (Scott, 1992).

It is important to evaluate, not only to assess the effect-iveness of any given campaign, but also to monitor progress; to measure impact; to maximise cost-efficiency; to share experience and, ultimately, it is an essential planning tool. The HIV/AIDS field is a particularly sensitive area. Data can often be manipulated or misinterpreted because it is a political as well as a social problem and one that highlights moral and ethical issues. By its nature 'evaluation is never a neutral and objective activity' (Aggleton and Moody, 1992). Thus particular attention must be given to the reasons for evaluation and the selection of methodology.

Very often the target setting for HIV/AIDS is given to those problems which are measurable but, as Johnson argues (Health of the Nation, 1992), setting targets for risk reduction and monitoring long-term risk behaviour is required. However, it is hard to measure outcome and behaviour change. It depends on what is being measured and for whom and any health-related behaviour cannot be seen in isolation from the individual's situation and circumstances. 'It is a mistake to focus on outcomes as separate entities for, unless an understanding is developed of the context in which health promotion takes place and the processes through which this work is carried out, even if seemingly positive outcomes are identified, there may be no means of explaining how they arose or how they can be reproduced' (Scott, 1992).

Holland and Fullerton (1995) state that evaluations make claims about the effects of interventions but this does little to establish effectiveness. They undertook a study to assess the effectiveness of 886 HIV/AIDS health promotion and education interventions. There were 114 reports of evaluations and these were studied by the authors for effectiveness and sound methodology. Five (33%) of the methodologic-ally sound studies were judged effective by authors and 3 (20%) by reviewers. Authors judged 33% of the flawed studies effective compared to 9% for reviewers. The largest difference between authors and reviewers for the flawed studies was that 43% were considered unclear by reviewers because of methodological problems and/or lack of necessary information. Overall, there was 54% agreement between authors and reviewers on effectiveness and in 6% of cases some agreement as to some effect; in 16% of cases authors said the intervention was effective and the reviewers disagreed, and in 21% of cases the reviewers judged the intervention to be unclear or ineffective when the authors' view was that it was partially effective.

According to Holland and Fullerton (1995), randomised control trials (RCTs) are the only effective and reliable way of establishing effectiveness of different types of intervention. Comparing the pre and post intervention measures against themselves, rather than a control population, provides inadequate data. They argue that 'it is the very complexity and multiplicity of factors influencing health attitudes and behaviours that strengthens the case for properly designed RCTs'. RCTs have been favoured by the medical profession in situations where there is uncertainty about whether a treatment or programme works. However, the urgency of the AIDS epidemic and the moral and ethical issues involved have meant that the 'lack of time justified lack of evaluation, and the 'unethics' of withholding from anyone something that might work functioned to dilute even further the gaol of establishing effective ways of tackling the progress or spread of the disease' (Holland and Fullerton, 1995).

Outcome measures, therefore, have been limited because of the lack of evidence that could have been supplied by RCTs. This, coupled with the pressure from management for interventions to supply information relevant to particular audits and the gap between research and policy and the inappropriate decisions made by policy makers, despite the findings of sound policies, have led to major obstacles in limiting the spread of HIV and AIDS. It is not just the prevention initiatives that need to be looked at for effectiveness in promoting sexual health, but also the context in which they are being provided. Often, there is a conflict between prevention and cure and management and funding, and evaluation is often used as the tool with which to battle this out (Scott, 1992).

Evaluation needs to be seen in the context of a whole range of aspects. It must reflect a consideration of the individual, future funding, ongoing support mechanisms for clients, workers and agencies, as well as being a tool to measure effectiveness. As Holland/Fullerton demonstrate, problems that have arisen within the field of HIV/AIDS health promotion have been through design fault (choice of methodology), lack of consensus about the choice of appropriate outcome targets, the huge variety of possible evaluation outcome measures, eg. the biological outcomes, behavioural outcomes, reduction of risk behaviours, protective behaviours and psychological outcomes. Added to this is the complication of measuring outcomes when the HIV incubation period is so long.

From the variety of evaluation outcome measures mentioned, it is easy to see how multidisciplinary the field of HIV/AIDS is. Therefore, the variety of ideologies and understandings attending the professional discipline (medical, psychological, management) are also great. The goals are shared, but there are many differing angles, such as 'to improve local people's knowledge of HIV/AIDS' or 'to reduce the spread of HIV infection in the local population' (Scott, 1992). Is the prevention programme to assess the potential saving of life by: raising awareness in the whole population or in a certain subgroup in the prevention of the spread of HIV, or in reducing discrimination by changing society's attitudes that, in turn, could improve people's quality of life and enable them to function within the community (Godfrey and Tolley, 1992)? Measuring quantity of life (number of life years) and quality of life is itself subjective.

Health promotion, in terms of HIV/AIDS, is sometimes evaluated in terms of behaviour change. More often than not this is what is required by the funders. The US Panel on the Evaluation of AIDS Interventions recommended behavioural measures as the primary outcome for most AIDS intervention programmes (Coyle: cited by Holland and Fullerton, 1995). Seroconversion rates are too problematic to measure because of the length of incubation and the use of this outcome measure requires large sample sizes.

As Holland and Fullerton (1995) point out 'a trial taking HIV infection as the outcome measure and using favourable assumptions (50% decrease in new infections due to the programme, 5% baseline seroconversion rate and 70% follow-up rate) would require recruitment of over 2500 injecting drug users' (School of Public Health and Institute for Health Policy Studies, 1993 cited in Holland and Fullerton, 1995). They also argue that 'the use of behavioural measures as 'proxy' indicators of the likelihood of infection requires a sound understanding, based on careful prior mapping, of the relationships between individual behaviours and the chance of acquiring HIV.' Scott (1992) argues that the relationship between knowledge, beliefs and behaviour is weak and using behaviour change as the central activity on which to focus HIV health promotion is limited. 'It is simply unrealistic to develop a yardstick for behaviour in the context of HIV/AIDS and then use it to assess everyone's progress . . . We must learn not to use common-sense categories and labels to tidy up the messiness and variety of everyday life' (Scott, 1992).

Critique of evaluation

Health promotion has been under the spotlight to reduce and control the spread of HIV. Pressure is being put on health workers to gain quantifiable, empirical evidence to assess the effectiveness of HIV prevention. Because HIV is a complex social issue as well as a disease, outcome-focused, goal-orientated evaluation in this context, often raises more questions of uncertainty, since it does not constitute a purely scientific problem. A good example is condom use and safer sex. This has been central to many health education campaigns and measured according to the uptake of condom-related behaviour.

However, as seen by the data produced by Holland *et al* (1992), condom use is linked to meanings and understandings that cannot easily be measured and to the existence of male control (Scott, 1992). Outcome measures, recording the number of times condoms are used, cannot guarantee condom use in the future or the complexities of negotiating their use. It is these hidden influences which need to be analysed and understood in order to promote effective HIV/AIDS health promotion (Scott, 1992). 'Poor measurement is worse than no measurement and, rather than being exact and scientific, a focus on outcome alone is likely to produce shallow results based on inadequate and superficial analysis' (Scott, 1992).

The need for secure resources and the competition for funds between the fields of prevention, treatment and research makes evaluation particularly important especially as estimates of HIV infection have been lower than predicted (Godfrey and Tolley, 1992). 'Early projections of HIV infection rates overestimated the numbers of AIDS cases in Britain, largely because behaviour change among gay men led to fewer cases than expected' (McEwan and Bhopal, 1991).

Predictions are difficult to make and for these to be useful, data on sexual behaviour of the population at risk, changes in sexual behaviour over time and the relationship between HIV infection and disease and the length of time it takes to develop AIDS are needed (Wellings *et al*, 1994). 'Efforts to mount effective public health education campaigns, to predict the likely extent and pattern of the spread of HIV and to plan services for those affected, have all been hampered by the absence of reliable data on sexual behaviour' (Wellings *et al*, 1994). The aim of the Sexual Behaviour in Britain Study carried out by the National Survey of Sexual Attitudes and Lifestyles was to provide data that would increase the understanding of the transmission patterns of HIV and assist in the selection of appropriate and effective health education strategies for epidemic control. They argue that preventative intervention needs an understanding of patterns of human sexuality in order to design effective interventions and advice on risk reduction (Wellings *et al*, 1994). This is backed up by Johnson (Department of Health, 1992) who argues that targets for HIV and AIDS have floundered largely on the problems of assessing the rate of spread of HIV in Britain. This is a result of both limited epidemiological data and a lack of baseline population estimates of risk behaviour, which are necessary to define the size of behaviour change required to control the epidemic.

The problem of risk behaviour and of understanding how to modify such action is central to the prevention and control of HIV/AIDS. However, as discussed, finding an outcome measure to assess the effectiveness of such initiatives is difficult, when examining health behaviour and the complex issues that make behaviour change problematic. Added to this, is the difficulty of attributing changes to a particular education programme. Assessing effectiveness of sexual health promotion is, therefore, difficult to prove because of the lack of data and concrete evidence to back up such claims. However, the challenge of HIV/AIDS has clarified many weaknesses, imbalances and inconsistencies in past health promotion efforts, but the WHO projects that the decade of the 1990s will provide greater pressures, expectations and opportunities for HIV/AIDS health promotion to take place. Despite the conflict and lack of consensus regarding the meaning and intended outcomes of sexual health initiatives, this should not preclude or diminish the importance and significance health promotion can play in the prevention of HIV/AIDS.

References

Adler M (1995) *ABC of Sexually Transmitted Diseases*, 3rd edn. British Medical Journal, London

Aggleton P, Moody D (1992) Monitoring and evaluation HIV/AIDS health education and health promotion. In: Aggleton P *et al*, eds. *Does It Work*. Health Education Authority, London

Aggleton P, Tyrer P (1994) Sexual health. In: Aggleton P *et al*, eds. *Learning About AIDS*, 2nd edn. Churchill Livingstone, Edinburgh: 72–88

Alcorn K, ed (1996) *AIDS Reference Manual*. NAM Publications, London

Bloor M (1995) A user's guide to contrasting theories of HIV related risk behaviour. In: Gabe J, ed. *Medicine, Health and Risk: Sociological Approaches*. Blackwell Scientific, Oxford

Cohen M, Chwalow J (1994) The Health Belief Model — always, sometimes or never useful in guiding HIV/AIDS prevention. In: Friedrick D, Heckmann W, eds. *AIDS in Europe — The Behavioural Aspect: Determinants of Behaviour Change*, vol 4. Rosch-Buch, Hallstadt

Department of Health (1992) *The Health of the Nation: A Strategy for Health in England*. HMSO, London

Friedrich L, Knox M, Boaz T, Dow M (1994) HIV risk factors for persons with serious mental illness. *Comm Ment Health J* **30**(6): 551–63

Godfrey C, Tolley K (1992) An economic approach to the evaluation of HIV/AIDS health education programmes. In: Aggleton P *et al*, eds. *Does it Work*. Health Education Authority, London

Holland J *et al* (1992) Pressure, resistance, empowerment: young women and the negotiation of safer sex. In: Aggleton P *et al*, eds. *AIDS: Rights and Reason*. Falmer Press, London

Holland J, Fullerton D (1995) Establishing the effectiveness of behavioural interventions to prevent HIV: some trials and tribulations. In: Friedrick D, Heckman W, eds. *Aids in Europe — The Behavioural Aspect: Determinants of Behaviour Change*, vol 4. Rosch-Buch, Hallstadt

Johnson A (1991) HIV/AIDS. In: *The Health of the Nation*. British Medical Journal, London

Kickbusch I (1994) Introduction: Tell me a story. In: Pederson A, O'Neill M, Rootman I, eds. *Health Promotion in Canada: Provincial, National and International Perspectives*. W B Saunders, Toronto

Mann S *et al* (1996) Pelvic inflammatory disease. *Int J STD AIDS* **7**: 315–21

McEwan R, Bhopal RL (1991) *HIV/AIDS Health Promotion for Young People: A Review of Theory, Principles and Practice*, Paper 12. Health Education Authority. HMSO, London

McHaffie H (1993) Improving awareness. *Nurs Times* **89**(18): 29–31

Pye K, Kapila W (1990) *AIDS Programme: Evaluation of AIDS Health Promotion Programmes: Concepts and The Cambridge Study*, Paper 7, Health Education Authority. HMSO, London

Scott S (1992) Evaluation may change your life, but it won't solve all your problems. In: Aggleton P *et al*, eds. *Does It Work*. Health Education Authority. HMSO, London

Scott S, Freeman R (1995) Prevention as a problem of modernity: the example of HIV/AIDS. In: Gabe J, ed. *Medicine, Health and Risk: Sociological Approaches*. Blackwell Scientific, Oxford

Smith A, Jacobson B, eds (1988) *The Nation's Health: A Strategy for the 1990s*. The Kings Fund, London

Tones B (1981) Health education: prevention or subversion? *R Soc Health J* **3**: 413–6

Wellings K *et al* (1994) *Sexual Behaviour in Britain*. Penguin, Harmondsworth

World Health Organization (1986) *Ottawa Charter for Health Promotion*. WHO, Geneva

12
Sexuality and sexual health: towards a dynamic nursing curriculum

Matthew V Morrissey and Shirley Crouch

Introduction

> *'I found it most difficult to cope with the men who drew sexual inferences as you did what you had to do. That made it very difficult. If you had somebody who played the game and went along with you it made it a lot easier. If you had someone who laid back there and leered at you and made comments about how enjoyable it was, that made it much more difficult'*
>
> (Lawler, 1991).

Clearly nurses maintain a fragile context of nursing practice when they perform body care for others which breaks many normal social rules about touch, body exposure, sexuality and sexual behaviour. The issue of sexuality education is very much on the political agenda in healthcare education (Schwartz, 1996: Waterhouse, 1996; McAlonan, 1996). Sexuality is an important aspect of care in a variety of settings with clients of all ages and most medical diagnosis, for example breast cancer (Baggs and Karch, 1987; Young, 1987; Nosek, 1996; Whipple *et al*, 1996; Lugton, 1997). Not only do nurses have to deal with many awkward and sensitive situations, they also need to maintain professional boundaries while respecting the needs of clients to express their sexuality. Education about sexuality and sexual health requires understanding of the work of nurses in practice. It is important to help nurses to develop effective methods of communication in the area of sexuality and sexual health promotion.

Creating a dynamic nursing curriculum requires an appreciation of the importance of sexuality within and outside of healthcare (Grigg, 1997; Tapp, 1997; Yarber and Torabi, 1997; Morrissey and Rivers, 1998). It is also vital that partnerships are formed so that educators and clinicians can develop a structure which can be applied to everyday nursing practice. The development of education in this area is important for all healthcare workers and a multi-professional approach is clearly needed (Kerr and Gasgoigne, 1996). There is also a need for the nurse educator to gain experience in using and creating more student-centred approaches in the teaching of sexuality and health. Traditional teaching methods have tended to focus on information rather than guiding the student nurse in practice. It is now understood that psychological and social issues are also important in relation to sexuality (Bruni, 1997; Kelly, 1997).

It is now clear that health professionals, particularly nurses, have much to contribute in relation to health education and sexual health over the life cycle, particularly in adolescence (Yarber and Torabi, 1997; Lugton, 1997). Respecting the rights and dignity of clients is an important aspect of care. Dealing with sensitive issues requires the development of a dynamic nursing curriculum with a clear foundation for the development of supportive policies on sexuality and sexual health in practice. This chapter examines how, using a model (Mims-Swenson Sexual Health Model), a curriculum can provide a basis for learning which can be directly related to the practice and development of nursing in sexuality and sexual health.

Sexual health

Purdie (1996) believes that most people learn about sexuality from their peers. How to be attractive to potential partners and how to function safely in sexual relationships. Personal development and self-awareness are essential in the effective functioning of individuals in their sexual relationships. These issues are encompassed in the values of Maddock (1976) who describes sexual health as an individual having cognitive knowledge about sexual phenomena, developing a degree of self-awareness about their own attitudes towards sex and sexuality, a well-developed, useable value system that provides input into sexual decisions and some degree of emotional comfort and stability in relation to the sexual activities in which the individual and others engage. These issues should be considered if a curriculum model is to be dynamic and effectively meet the aims of educating health workers in the area of sexuality. If there is not an appropriate medium for people to learn about sexuality, sexual health development of the individual can be restricted.

Concept of sexual health and the role of the nurse

The sexual health of the individual develops on a continuum from childhood to elderly adulthood. Many factors influence sexuality and personal development. Developmental issues focus on human development, psychological processes and events during various stages of the life cycle and the events that might positively or adversely affect that development. The individual needs to make adjustments at different times in life, identifying new requisites derived from many different situations and relationships.

A deviation from sexual health exists for people who are ill, injured, have specific forms of pathology, including defects and disabilities which may result in biological dysfunction or structure, in physical functioning or in behaviour and habits of what is deemed usual 'sexual requisites'. (McAlonan, 1996; McCarthy, 1996; Whipple *et al*, 1996; Ryan, 1997). Healthcare professionals and nurses clearly have a central role in treating such health problems and helping clients readjust as well as possible to physical impairments. Sexuality includes more than a biological response; it involves communication, forming relationships, expressions of self, physical contact, affection and love. How we learn is very much a social experience which may effect the way we react to individual situations (Bandura, 1986). Affirmative education is important in the area of sexuality for healthcare workers given that many individuals grow up with negative views of their own sexuality and the sexuality of others.

Health professionals need to understand how to respond to the clients in their care. The individual's sexuality is affected, for example, after surgery, during intervention to reproductive organs, rape, sexual abuse and the ending of a relationship through failure or the death of a partner. In many of these situations, the nurse has an important role to play within the multidisciplinary team and she/he needs to be knowledgeable and skilled in her/his interventions.

Sexuality and nurse education

A study by the World Health Organization in 1973 indicated that little sexuality content was being taught in medical and nursing schools throughout the world, and this organisation encouraged schools to add more information on sexuality (Mace *et al*, 1974; World Health Organization, 1975). Browning and Lewis (1976) published a text on the nursing implications of human sexuality in 1973. A year later sexuality was included as an area warranting nursing assessment by the medical-surgical division of the American Nursing Association. By the mid 1970s, numerous references to sexuality had appeared in nursing journals (Bullough and Seidi, 1974; Mims *et al*, 1976) and several research studies were published about nursing knowledge, attitudes and education related to sexuality (Payne, 1976; Lief and Payne, 1975). Sexuality was included in general nursing texts beginning in the late seventies (Cambell, 1978). Sexuality was increasingly incorporated into nurse education, research, and publications during the 1980s (Frazer *et al*, 1982; Wilson and Williams, 1988). Currently, most nursing texts include some content on sexuality (Carpenito, 1995; Phillips *et al*, 1995) and most nursing courses include content on sexuality integrated throughout the curriculum, or as a separate course or module (Katzman and Katzman, 1987).

Several recent publications continue to document the lack of appropriate preparation of healthcare workers, including nurses, for the teaching of sexuality to clients (Waterhouse, 1996; Purdie, 1996). This lack of preparation cannot be blamed only on medical and nursing education, but also on the inherent beliefs and values that every individual brings to education and the workplace. Research has shown that nurses are reluctant to discuss sexuality issues with clients, much of this reluctance being due to the lack of knowledge and ability to embrace such personal issues (Kantz et al, 1990). Due to lack of clear guidelines or policies in practice, there is a real fear of ethical dilemmas arising as a result of lack of training and education in relation to sexuality and healthcare. Confidence in teaching and practice in relation to sexuality is not simply due to accumulating knowledge but how comfortable a teacher is with his/her own sexuality and that of others (Grigg 1997).

Rather than traditional teaching methods, the use of workshops has shown that, when healthcare professionals and nurses have opportunities to explore sexuality issues, a more positive approach is adopted (Frazer, 1982; Matocha and Waterhouse, 1993; Kantz et al, 1990). Previous literature has identified the need for educators to have opportunities to discuss sexuality and to develop appropriate learning experiences that do not impinge on the client's privacy and dignity (Purdie, 1996; Morrissey and Rivers, 1998). At the same time, teaching sexuality and sexual health needs to be developed from the experience level to an advanced level and this is the focus of the Mims Swenson Sexual Health Model.

A sexual health model

There are a number of advantages in using a sexual health model to guide teaching and learning. The Mims-Swenson Sexual Health Model (1980) was adapted from the P-LI-SS-IT model (Anon, 1976) and both provide frameworks for self-assessment, intervention and planning of practitioner education for the promotion of sexual health. The Mims-Swenson Sexual Health Model consists of four ascending levels of analysis (life experience, basic, intermediate and advanced) covering knowledge, attitudes and nursing practice. Morrissey and Rivers (1998) have developed a curriculum, based on this model, for the education of nurses on the needs of lesbian, gay or bisexual individuals.

There are many individuals who are unable to attain sexual health because of physical, psychological, social, economic and political prejudices, or through sensory and cognitive impairment. Views on sexuality are influenced by past experiences, family, friends, the legal system, government policy and the media. All people need to be given the opportunity to make sense of their bodies and feelings throughout their lifespan. This being the case, healthcare workers have a role to play in facilitating this opportunity.

In the past, according to Waterhouse (1996), nurses have underestimated the needs of people in their care when it comes to issues of sexuality, and it has been suggested that they have not, as a matter of course, addressed the issue of sexuality in their practice. We can assume from this that nurse education does not effectively prepare practitioners to deal appropriately with the personal concerns of clients and sexuality.

The Mims-Swenson Sexual Health Model

The Mims-Swenson Sexual Health Model is used in conjunction with a humanistic approach which recognises that an individual's sexuality evolves throughout the lifespan. It acknowledges that there are several ascending levels in the acquisition of these abilities. Not only the clients that nurses care for are at different stages of development in their life's continuum, but so, too, are the staff who deliver their care, and this should be acknowledged.

Morrissey and Rivers (1998) suggest that nurses should only take on these activities at different stages of their own development. This is because it is acknowledged that sexuality is a very fragile entity and can easily be affected or damaged by inappropriate, or ill-informed interventions. It can be seen that the authors utilise the Mims-Swenson Model (1980), but emphasise the need for reassessment at each ascending level. During the assessment phase, it is important that the student reflects on sexual issues to identify beliefs and values (Crouch, 1997). Initially, it is important for the student to identify current knowledge surrounding sexuality and to reflect on and explore issues to do with sexual experiences and fantasies. They should explore issues to do with their own personal identity, reflect on how personal views might impact on care and identify areas for exploration and exposition. The reflective tool will assist the student to identify areas for exploration and exposition within a framework of mutual disclosure. Through discussion and disclosure, students should then become aware of how their personal beliefs, values and life experiences might impact on their care delivery in a confidential setting.

The Mims-Swenson Sexual Health Model consists of four ascending levels of analysis addressing both attitudes and knowledge in nursing practice: (1) life experience, (2) basic, (3) intermediate and

(4) advanced. As nurses progress through each level in turn, they are not only required to build upon their basic counselling and interactive skills, but examine more closely both personal and societal attitudes towards sexuality. The ethos underlying each of the ascending levels is outlined.

1. Life experience

At the first level in this model nurses are asked to focus upon the way in which both destructive and intuitively helpful behaviours are moulded by society's many taboos, myths and the stereotypic responses which surround sexual behaviour.

2. Basic level

At this level, individual perceptions, attitudes and cognitions are explored to raise the level of personal awareness. The basic level emphasises the point that all health professionals need to address their own, often long-held values and attitudes relating to sexuality, in order to provide an effective therapeutic relationship with clients. Mims and Swenson (1980) argue that, only through raising levels of personal awareness can health professionals develop a balanced viewpoint, which recognises their own value system, but, simultaneously, allows them to be accepting, or at least non-judgmental about the values of others.

3. Intermediate level

The intermediate level focuses upon both the method and process of communication between the nurse and the client. In this section particular attention is paid to ways of communicating to the client that their own sexual concerns are important and integral components of health. Furthermore, it gives guidance and instruction to the nurse on ways of providing direct and accurate information on sexuality to the client group concerned. For example, nurses working with clients, who have undergone mastectomies, hysterectomies and other invasive surgical procedures, should facilitate discussion of sexual concerns related to living and adapting to these changes for both clients and their partners (Waterhouse, 1996). Other important aspects to care include adjusting to disability and the effects of medication, particularly on clients with mental health problems. At this level, it is imperative that the nurse feels confident in his/her knowledge about human sexuality and is able to relay this information to the client through the use of appropriate communication skills and self-awareness. Students are required to take part in extensive workshop activities and role play. They should practice applying the knowledge and skills which they have acquired in a safe forum. Such activities might include explicit physical or psychological care and the use of language that is easily understood by the client.

4. Advanced level

At this level, the nurse's role is to provide suggestions, education programmes, therapy and, where feasible, conduct research on sexual health. Graduate education is the key to success at this level, enabling the health professional to design or revise educational programmes, engage in sex therapy and conduct research on sexual issues. Through education and research (which will inform education at all four levels), nurses will be able to practice and develop new skills which will effectively address the sexual health issues of the client during care (Smith, 1993).

Each level needs to be evaluated by the student to identify the processes and skills involved, their effectiveness and other learning goals that are personally required. Although the Mims-Swenson Sexual Health Model has been shown to be a useful conceptual framework in research (Smith, 1993), it has yet to be applied to training and evaluation for professional practice. However, its predecessor, the P-LI-SS-T Model developed by Anon (1976), has been applied to practice with respect to dealing with sexual issues and it has achieved some positive results (Cooley and Yeomans, 1986). According to Cooley and Yeomans, the application of the P-LI-SS-T Model to nurse education would allow up to 70% of clients to receive an appropriate level of support and counselling from the practice nurse through the utilisation of the first three levels of intervention (gained on undergraduate and pre-registration courses). Only 30% of clients would require specialist counselling from health professionals with a graduate education background. Unfortunately, such models do not guarantee that the personally held beliefs of nurses will change, and it has been suggested recently that, in the case of HIV/AIDS, attitudes persist even after extensive training (Tierney, 1995). These attitudes include fear and loathing of those infected with HIV (Green and Platt, 1997). It is clear, however, that the incorporation of a programme of sexual health education into nurse training encourages a much more effective client-orientated service within the caring professions. It has been suggested that nurses have not, as a matter of course, addressed the issue of sexuality in their practice and nurse education rarely prepares the practitioner to deal effectively with the personal concerns of clients (Waterhouse, 1996; Grigg, 1997). The authors suggest that a course based on the Mims-Swenson Sexual Health Model may enhance both the delivery and development of diploma and undergraduate nurse education in relation to human sexuality (this interpretation of the model acknowledges that nurse education needs to be developed at both postgraduate and advanced level). Its purpose is to offer nurses the opportunity to develop and put into practice basic skills in dealing with sexuality. It is important that a variety of non-traditional teaching methods are introduced, which enhance the teaching of sexuality (Haignere et al, 1996). Methods may include: case presentations, role play and experiential workshops where students can explore personal and professional attitudes, beliefs and values surrounding sexuality in a safe and non-judgmental environment.

Caution is needed. We must not assume such education is a 'one off'. The Mims-Swenson Sexual Health Model as proposed here also emphasises the importance of development. To be a sexual counsellor is a highly skilled role, which requires extensive knowledge and training, and nurses should not attempt this unless they have acquired these skills.

Mulleady (1992) focuses on the issue that workers should 'examine their own attitudes' and modify their prejudices to enable them to talk to clients about sex. Purdie (1996) suggests that this is a fragile argument, because it implies that if we attempt to modify our attitudes, it automatically follows that we will be competent to counsel individuals on sexual matters. Mulleady's argument does not acknowledge the skills, knowledge and training required before sexual counselling should be undertaken. To disregard this trivialises sexuality, as it implies that anyone can help others if they stand back from their own beliefs. Education and training enables health workers to internalise and intellectualise the issues. This should then expand health workers' abilities and intellect, allowing them to overcome their fears and ignorance. However, before this development can take place, professionals have to be honest about their own sexual desires, needs and fantasies and be comfortable with them if they hope to be of use to those with a different sexual orientation. Prejudice surrounding sexual issues is a barrier towards effective communication. To help improve care of all patients, nurse education needs to address the knowledge base and skills of nurse educators in the teaching of sexual health to students. They should avoid the presumption that patients become asexual when in need of care, acknowledging that sexuality is important and multidimensional. Patients/clients are not simply ticked off on a care plan or excluded, stereotypes and myths need to be dispelled and prejudices and preconceptions challenged.

Nurses need to be presented with positive and realistic images of sexuality and sexual health, relationships and sexual life styles. Beliefs and values and the influence of perpetuating prejudices need to be examined. It must also be appreciated that the attitudes of healthcare workers are very much influenced by their socialisation (Eliason, 1993). Such a process of education begins at school, in the primary and secondary education of children (Lammers, 1996; Tapp et al, 1997; Yarber and Torabi, 1997). Education and teaching about human relationships are important and must be sensitively applied to the needs of children so that they can grow up with a positive view of themselves and their sexuality. Much of sex education has focused on safer sex. Yet what is really required in our society is responsible and loving relationships. Although sex and sexuality may hold the central spotlight and be greatly desired and worshipped, the ultimate human need is love.

References

Anon J (1976) The P-LI-SS-IT Models. *J Sex Educ Ther* **2**: 1–15

Baggs JG, Karch AM (1987) Sexual counselling of women with coronary heart disease. *Heart Lung* **16**: 154–9

Bandura A (1986) *Social Foundations of Thought and Action: A Social Cognitive Theory*. Prentice-Hall, New Jersey

Browning M, Lewis (1976) *Human Sexuality: Human Implications*. American Journal of Nursing, New York

Bruni N (1997) The nurse educator as teacher: exploring the construction of the 'reluctant instructor'. *Nurs Inq* **4**(1): 34–40

Bullough VL, Seidi A (1987) Attitudes on sexuality in nursing texts today and yesterday. *Hol Nurs Pract* **1**: 84–92

Cambell C (1978) Nursing Diagnosis and Intervention in Nursing Practice. John Wiley, Chichester and New York

Carpenito LJ (1995) *Nursing Diagnosis: Application to Clinical Practice*, 6th edn. JB Lippincott, Philadelphia

Cooley M, Yeomans A (1986) Sexual and reproductive issues for women with Hodgkin's Disease. Application of the P-LI-SS-IT model. *Cancer Nurs* **9**(5): 248–55

Crouch SE (1997) Reflection on Beliefs and Values Regarding Sexuality. Unpublished reflective tool

Eliason MJ (1993) Cultural diversity in nursing care: The lesbian, gay or bisexual persons. *J Transcult Nurs* **5**(1): 14–20

Frazer J (1982) Impact of a human sexuality workshop on the sexual attitudes and knowledge of nursing students. *J Nurs Educ* **21**(3): 6–13

Frazer J, Albert M, Smith J, *et al* (1982) Impact of human sexuality workshop on the sexual attitudes and knowledge of nursing students. *J Nurs Educ* **21**. 252–5

Glover J (1985) *Human Sexuality in Nursing Care*. Croom Helm, London

Green G, Platt S (1997) Fear and loathing in healthcare settings reported by people with HIV. *Sociol Health Illness* **19**(1): 70–92

Grey A (1993) *Speaking of Sex — The Limits of Language*. Cassell Publication, London

Grigg E (1997) Guidelines for teaching about sexuality. *Nurse Educ Today* **17**(1): 62–6

Haignere CS, Culhane JF, Basley CM, Legos P (1996) Teachers receptiveness and comfort teaching sexuality education and using non-traditional teaching strategies. *J School Health* **66**(4): 140–4

Kantz DD, Dickey CA, Stevens MN (1990) Using research to identify why nurses do not meet established sexuality nursing care standards. *J Nurs Qual Ass* **4**(3): 69–78

Katzman EM, Katzman LS (1987) Outcomes of sexuality course in nursing education. *J Sex Educ Ther* **13**: 33–6

Kelly E (1997) Development of strategies to identify the learning needs of baccalaureate nursing students. *J Nurs Educ* **36**(4): 156–62

Kelly JA, Lawrence St JS, Hood HV, Smith S, Cook DJ (1988) Nurses attitudes towards Aids. *J Contin Educ Nurs* **19**: 78–83

Kerr DL, Gasgoigne JL (1996) Getting to know generation X: health education for the thirteenth generation. *J Health Educ* **27**(5): 268–76

Lammers JV (1996) The effects of curriculum on student health behaviours: a case study of the growing health curriculum on the health behaviours of eight grade students. *J Health Educ* **27**(5): 278–85

Lawler J (1991) *Behind the Screens Nursing, Somology, and the Problem of the Body*. Churchill Livingstone, Edinburgh

Lief HI, Payne T (1975) Sexuality-knowledge and attitudes. *Am J Nurs* **75**: 2026–9

Lugton J (1997) Health visitor support for patients with breast cancer, part two. *Nurs Stand* **11**(35): 34–8

Mace DR, Brauerman RH, Burton J (1974) *Teaching of Human Sexuality in Schools for Health Professionals*. World Health Organization, Geneva

Maddock J (1976) Sexual health: an enrichment and treatment programme. In: Olson DH, ed. *Treating Relationships*. Graphic Publishers, London

Matocha LK, Waterhouse JK (1993) Current nursing practice related to sexuality. *Res Nurs Health* **16**: 371–8

McAlonan S (1996) Improving sexual rehabilitation services: the patients perspective. *Am J Occ Ther* **50**(10): 826–34

McCarthy M (1996) The sexual support needs of people with learning disabilities: a profile of those referred for sex education. *Sexual Disabil* **14**(4): 265–79

Mims FH, Brown L, Lubow R (1976) Human sexuality course evaluation. *Nurs Res* **25**: 187–91

Mims FH, Swenson M (1980) *Sexuality: A Nursing Perspective*. McGraw Hill: New York

Morrissey M, Rivers I (1998) Applying the Mims-Swenson Sexual Health Model to nurse education: A focus on sexuality and healthcare. *Nurse Educ Today* **18**: 488–95

Mulleady G (1992) *Counselling Drug Users About HIV and AIDS*. Blackwell Scientific, Oxford

Nosek MA (1996) Wellness among women with physical disabilities. *Sexual Disabil* **14**(3): 183–90

Payne T (1976) Sexuality of nurses: correlations of knowledge, attitudes and behaviour. *Nurs Res* **25**:187–91

Phillips WJ, Cassmeyer VL, Sands JK, Lehman MK (1995) *Medical-surgical Nursing: Concepts and Practice*. Mosby, St Louis

Platzer H (1993) Nursing care of gay and lesbian patients. *Nurs Stand* **7**(17): 35–7

Purdie H (1996) Management of sexuality in a mental health setting. *Nurs Stand* **11**(12): 47–50

Rowan J (1989) *The Hemmed God. Feminism and Health as Wounding and Healing*. Routledge, London

Ryan S (1997) How rheumatoid arthritis affects patients and families. *Nurs Times* **93**(18): 48–9

Schwartz IM (1996) Sexuality education, HIV/AIDS education, and contraceptive use during initial coitus as perceived among female students: a comparison between the United States and Sweden. *J Health Educ* **27**(3): 156–64

Smith GB (1993) Homophobia and attitudes towards gay men and lesbians by psychiatric nurses. *Arch Psychiatr Nurs* **7**(6): 377–84

Tapp MK, Galer-Unti RA, Bailey KC (1997) Evaluation of trained teachers' implementation of a sex education curriculum. *J Health Educ* **28**(2): 103–8

Tierney AJ (1995) HIV/AIDS knowledge, attitudes and education of nurses: a review of the research. *J Clin Nurs* **4**(1): 13–21

Waterhouse J (1996) Nursing practice related to sexuality: a review and recommendations. *Nurs Times Res* **1**(6): 412–8

Whipple B, Richards E, Tepper M, Komisaruk BR (1996) Sexual response in women with complete spinal cord injury. *Sexual Disabil* **14**(3): 191–201

Wilson ME, Williams HA (1988) Oncology nurses' attitudes and behaviours related to sexuality of patients with cancer. *Oncol Nurs For* **15**: 49–52

World Health Organization (1975) *Education and Treatment in Human Sexuality: The Training of Health Professionals*. WHO, Geneva

Yarber WL, Torabi MR (1997) Impact of a theory based school HIV/STD curriculum on eight graders' attitudes and knowledge. *J Health Educ* **28**(2): 74–84

Young EW (1987) Sexual needs of psychiatric clients. *J Psychosoc Nurs* 25: 30–2

Appendix

Reflective tool to help students explore personal beliefs and values regarding sexuality, Crouch (1997)

What do you think and how do you define sexuality?	
What do you feel about:	
Lesbians?	
Gay men?	
Children?	
Adolescents?	
The middle-aged?	
The elderly?	
Expression of self?	
Where do you think these perceptions have come from?	
How do you respond to sexist comments?	
How do you respond to homophobic comments?	
Do you respond in the same way in the care environment?	
Do you assume that all patients in your care are heterosexual?	
Are allowances made to assume that some clients might be gay, ie. assessment, admission slips, next of kin, privacy?	
Do you know of any instances where 'care' has not been fully delivered because the nurse or health worker has felt uncomfortable with sexuality issues?	

Describe here: Would you be prepared to speak out where sexism or homophobia occurs in society? Are there any areas regarding sexuality that you would like to explore further?	

CONTACTS

If you need help, advice or assistance, contact one of these organisations

Organisations

AIDS Helpline Northern Ireland:
01232-326117
7.30pm–10pm, Monday–Friday

AIDS North
0191-232 2855
7pm–10pm, Wednesday and Friday. Otherwise a recorded message. For local AIDS helplines, look in your telephone book.

Association for Lesbian, Gay and Bisexual Psychologists (ALGBP)
PO Box 7534
London, NW1 0ZA

Association to Aid Sexual and Personal Relationships of People with a Disability (SPOD)
286 Camden Road
London, N7 0BE

Body Positive
51B Philbeach Gardens
London, SW6 9EB
Run by and for people who are HIV antibody positive. Provides support, help and advice.

British Association for Sexual and Marital Therapy
PO Box 62
Sheffield, S10 3TS

Brook Advisory Centres
223 Tottenham Court Road
London W1A 9AE
Clinics in various cities — they provide confidential advice on contraception, pregnancy, abortion and emotional and sexual problems for young people. Look in your telephone book under **Family Planning.**

DAWN (Drugs, Alcohol, Women, Nationally)
Omnibus Workspace
39/41 North Road
London, N7 9DP
Provides information, support and advice for women on drug use, and on HIV and AIDS.

Domestic Violence Intervention Project: Violence Prevention Programme
PO Box 2838
London, W6 9ZE
Tel: 0181 563 7983

Family Planning Association
27/35, Mortimer Street,
London, WC1M 7RJ
2–12 Pentonville Road
London, N1 9FP
Tel: 0171 837 5432
Helpline: 0171 837 4044
Information and education
0171 837 3034

6 Windsor Place,
Cardiff, CF1 3BX

113 University Street,
Belfast, BT7 1HP

4 Clifton Street
Glasgow, G3 7LA
Regional offices which will provide information on local FPA clinics. Clinics are run through the NHS and do not need a GP referral.

Feminist Library Resource and Information Centre
5 Westminster Bridge Road
London, SE1 7XW
Tel: 0171 928 7789

Friends and Families of Lesbians and Gays (FFLAG)
PO Box 153
Manchester, M60 1LP

Frontliners
52/54 Grays Inn Road
London, WC1X 8JU

    Run by and for people with AIDS and provides information, help and support.

The Haemophilia Society
123, Westminster Bridge Road
London, SE1 7HR

    For help and advice for haemophilia sufferers, their friends, partners and families.

Health Education Authority
Hamilton House
Mabledon Place
London, WC1H 9TX

    Provides a free resource list on AIDS which includes books, films, videos etc.

Institute of Psychosexual Medicine
11 Chandos Street
Cavendish Square
London, W1M 9DE

    Tel: 0171 580 0631

Kings Fund Library and Information Service (KFLIS)
11-13 Cavendish Square
London, W1M 0AN

    Tel: 0171 307 2568/9
    Fax: 0171 307 2805
    Email: libenq2@kehf.org.uk

London Lesbian and Gay Switchboard
    Tel: 0171 837 7324

London Lighthouse
111/117 Lancaster Road
London W11 1QT

    Provides support, help and advice on HIV and AIDS, with a residential unit for people with AIDS.

Mainliners
359 Old Kent Road
London, SE1

    Run by and for current and ex-drug users who are HIV positive, or have AIDS or AIDS-Related Complex. They provide help, support and information.

National AIDS Helpline:
0800-567123

    All calls are free, open 24 hours a day. Provides a confidential information and advice service on all aspects of HIV and AIDS.

National Childbirth Trust (NCT)
Alexandra House
Oldham Terrace
Acton
London, W3 6NH

    Tel: 0181 992 2616 (Administration)
    Helpline: 0181 992 8637 (Enquiries)
    Fax: 0181 992 5929

Pace: The Project for Advice, Counselling and Education
34 Hartham Road
London, N7 9JL

    Tel: 0171 700 1323
    Fax: 0171 609 4909

Positive Care in Obstetrics and Gynaecology (PCOG)
7 Princess Street
Oxford, OX4 1DD

    Tel: 01865 726755

Positive Partners
c/o Lorraine Ainscow, 10 Rathbone Place,
London W1

    A support group for partners who are HIV positive or have AIDS.

Pregnancy Advisory Service (PAS)
11-13 Charlotte Street
London, W1P 1HD

    Tel: 0171 637 8962

SCODA (Standing Conference on Drug Abuse)
1/4 Hatton Place
Hatton Garden
London, EC1N 8ND

    Provides information and advice to drug users on HIV and AIDS, including details of your nearest needle exchange.

Scottish AIDS Monitor (SAM)
PO Box 48,
Edinburgh, EH1 5SE

    Provides advice, information and help on all aspects of AIDS

Sex Education Forum
Tel: 0171 843 6000
> Monday–Friday
> Training and consultancy to schools

Sexual Health and STD clinics (VD)
> Advice is free and given in confidence. Look in the telephone book under 'Venereal Disease' or 'Sexually Transmitted Disease'. If you have difficulty call your nearest main hospital; ask your GP; telephone the Family Planning Information Service.

The Terence Higgins Trust
52/54 Grays Inn Road
London, WC1X 8JU
> Provides advice, information and help on all aspects of HIV and AIDS.
> Legal advice, for example insurance or employment rights

UKCP
167–169 Great Portland Street
London W1N 5FB
Tel: 0171 436 3002
Fax: 0171 436 3013

VISTEL 0800-521361
> 10am–10pm every day.

Cantonese: 0800-282446
> 6pm–10pm, Tuesdays

Hindi, Gujerati, Punjabi, Bengali and Urdu: 0800-282445
> 6pm-10pm, Wednesdays

Wellbeing — The Health Research Charity for Women and Babies
27 Sussex Place
Regent's Park
London, NW1 4SP
> Tel: 0171 262 5337
> Fax: 0171 724 7725
> Email: marystanton@wellbeing.org.uk

Welsh AIDS Campaign
PO Box 348
Cardiff, CF1 4LX
> Provides information and advice, and leaflets in English and Welsh.

Women's Health Information Centre
52 Featherstone Street
London, E1Y 8RT
> Provides information on women's health issues

Your GP
> For all medical problems.
> Remember that anything that you tell your GP will be included in your notes, and if they are asked for a report on your health for an insurance policy, or a mortgate, this information may prejudice your chances.

PUBLICATIONS

BSS, 252 Western Avenue
London, W3 6XJ
> *AIDS Now* — Price £1.00

AIDS and HIV:
Community Drug Project,
30 Manor Place, London, SE17 3BB
> *More Facts About AIDS Drug Users:*

NACAB Vision
Myddleton House
115 Pentonville Road
London, N1 9LZ
> Training video and Manual

Terence Higgins Trust,
52/54 Grays Inn Road,
London, WC1X 8JU
> *Safer Drug Use: A User's Guide*
> *A Positive Approach*:

PUBLICATIONS — coming soon

Central TV, Broad Street,
Birmingham, B1 2JP

Help, Thames Television, 164 Drummon Street
> *AIDS Help:*
> *Caring for People with HIV Infection:*

Welsh AIDS Campaign,
PO Box 348
Cardiff, CF1 4XI
> *AIDS — What it Means for Young People:*
> In English and Welsh

Guild Sound and Vision
6 Royce Road
Peterborough

VIDEOS AIDS Help:
70 minutes; five 10 minute episodes and four 5 minutes episodes. A series of programmes looking at various aspects of AIDS

Coming Soon:
Five 10 minute programmes aimed at young people.

Index

A

A sexual health model 228
abnormal 49, 64, 72
abnormal grief reaction 108
abstruse thought 40
abuse 78, 176
acquired immunodeficiency syndrome 87
activity of daily living 205
adjudicate 55
admission to hospital 175
adolescent pregnancy 127
adult survivors of sexual abuse 85
affirmative approach 106
affirmative therapy 67
agency policy 175
aggression 98, 116
AIDS 11, 15, 25, 31-32, 87, 99, 101, 104, 109, 166, 209-210, 212-214, 219, 221
AIDS epidemic 66, 219
AIDS Intervention programmes 220
AIDS sector 103
AIDS-related illness 34
alcohol abuse 106, 178
American Nursing Association 227
Amnesty International 103
animal behaviour 80
animal studies 79
animal-like drive 174
anthropologists 62
anxiety 119
Are preventive strategies empowering 210
Are you gay or straight 95
Aristophanes 96
Aristotle 19, 96
arousability 79
artificial and a fictitious unity 4
asexual 121, 160, 167, 190, 232
assertiveness 177
assessing sexual health needs of clients with schizophrenia 180
assessment phase 123, 229
assessment sheet 180
athletic ability 119
attitudes from our past 197
autonomy 209
aversion therapy 100
AVERT 99

B

Basic level 230
behaviour change 211
behavioural conformity 7
benchmarks 61
biological
    aspects 123
    determinism 78
    perspectives 76, 78
    phenomenon xiv
    sex 163
Biological or social: the problem of sexuality 160
biologically innate 81
biomedical model 214
bio-power 3-5, 14, 24
biopsychosocial model of childbirth 83
biopsychosocial phenomenon 76
bisexual clients 95
bisexual issues 66-67, 100
blame 210
body ideal 195
    positive 101
    presentation 193, 195
    reality 195
Bowlby 145
breadwinner 116
British Medical Journal 101
British Psychological Society 102
bullying 99
    in UK schools 98

C

cancer screening 106
care plan 180
categorisations 159-160
celebratory approach 39
censorship 166
chameleon concept 42
child abuse 138, 152-153
    protection workers 168
    sexual abuse 55, 138, 176
childbirth 75-76, 82, 86
childcare 163
childhood 115, 118, 122, 226
childhood imagery 146
child-rearing 88, 127, 139-143

child-rearing expert 127, 129, 139-142, 149, 151-152
Children's Act 135-136
Christian sexual values 17
citizenship cultures 20, 28
classification 159-160
Clinician philosophers 54
clinicians 182
closed-couple relationships 30
The Code of Conduct 198, 201
coercion 210
cognitive development 116
coitus in pregnancy 82
coming out 99
commodities 4, 22
common-sense 6-10, 12, 32, 33
communication skills 203
communications about sex 180
community barriers to sexual health promotion 212
community-based initiatives 211
concentration camps 100
concept of ourselves 192
concept of sexual health 45
and the role of the nurse 226
concept of sexuality 117
conception of despair 55
conceptual approach 42
conceptual clarity 55
condom use 220
consent 18
Constructing gender: constructing sexuality 77, 162
consumer 22
continental philosophy 44
contraceptive counselling 178
control 136-137, 141, 143, 150-153
coronary heart disease 115
correct practice 159
Council of Europe 102
counsellors 160, 182
Criminal Justice Act 131, 135-136
criminal offences 104
critique of evaluation 220
Cruisaid 101
cultural
conventions 7
definitions of gender 116
determinants 40
diversity 109
perspectives 76, 81
practices 83

D

Darwin 62
degrees of bisexuality 13
delay 216
denial 216
denial of sexuality 122
depression 106
desexualise 75
development of education 225
developmental disorder 103
developmental model of sexuality 77
deviants 10, 64
dignity 105
disability 205, 212
discourses of normality 160
discourses of sexuality 161
discrimination 104
    gay 65
    lesbian 65
discursive explosion 16
displacement 216
dissociation 86
diversity of healthcare xiii
domestic labour 163-164
domestic violence 106
dominant sexual order 20
domination 6
drive to consume 22
drug use 211
drugs and sexuality 174
duality of the mind/body 50
dynamic nursing curriculum xv, 225
dynamics of social interactions 216
dysphoria 70

E

early forced sexual intercourse 138
eastern philosophy 105
eastern religions 105
education xiii, 109, 177, 211
    and policies in practice 106
    and training 205
    for health professionals xiii
    interventions 218
    of children 122
    system 124
ego-dystonic homosexuality 66, 101
elderly adulthood 226
emergence 14
empirical assessment 47
    evidence 78
empowerment 177, 209-210, 215, 217
enlightenment 39, 159
epidemiological treatment 212

equal rights 102, 104
errors of superimposition 43
essentialist 8, 12, 160-162
    discourse 165
    opinion 14
ethical dilemmas 228
ethics 40
ethnic minority males 29
ethnocentric conclusions 7
ethnographers 62
Eugenic
    themes 163
    movement 162
evaluate current health promotion xvi
evaluation xv, 217-220
examine issues xvi
existentialism 44
experts 3, 9, 160
exploitation 176
explore the theoretical aspects xv
extramarital regulations 163
extrapyramidal side-effects 181

F

42nd Street 103
factory acts 163
False Memory Syndrome 144
family interactions 118
family planning services 115
female sexual response cycle 78
female sexuality 75-77
feminist 127, 148-149, 152
Firestone 144
Focus of the debate 209
folk devils 25
Foucault 44-45, 77, 160
freedom 41
Freud 8, 43-44, 46, 53, 63, 77, 116-117, 144, 150, 152, 174
fundamental view 121
funerals 105

G

Gai Pied 30
gay 95
    bathhouses 35
    doctors 29
    gene 8, 102
    issues 100
    liberation 101
    Liberation Front 101
    marriages 103
    media 24
    men 98

Pride Rally 29
relationship 66
rights movement 65
Times 29
gender
    confusion 70
    roles 116, 163
general practice 106
genetic engineering 102
genetic origins 66
geneticists 8
genital nature 118
GHA Survey Results 30
Gillick 134-135
good versus evil 41
graduate education 231
Greeks 96
group work 183
guidelines 178, 182
    for re-evaluating attitudes to sexuality 199

H

health attitudes 219
    education 214-215, 217
    education campaigns 220
    professionals 105
    promotion 214-215, 217-218, 220, 222
    risks 129-131
    threat 216
Health Belief Model 216
Health of the Nation 115, 130, 133, 209, 212
healthcare
    education 225
    policies 109
    professional 203, 227
    providers 200
    workers 174, 225
Hercules 96
heterosexual 6
    bias 107
    gene 8
hidden agenda 200
Hirschfeld 64
historical
    and contemporary overview of sexual health 43
    and psychological perspectives 76
    perspectives 76
    perspectives in the study of human sexuality 63
    processes 160

History, homosexuality and society 95
Hite Report 79
HIV 27-28, 32, 50, 87, 115, 175, 209-210, 212-215, 217, 219-220, 231
    health promotion 220
    incubation period 219
    infection 31, 33, 106, 209-210, 213-214, 216, 219-221
    infection rates 221
    intervention 215
    prevention 209-210, 215
    status 29
    test 32, 34
    transmission 25
    treatment 103
HIV/AIDS xv, 101, 106-107, 124, 177, 209, 212-213, 217-221, 231
    health promotion 210, 219, 221-222
    prevention 182
HIV-related
    illnesses 32
    risk behaviour 216
holism 205
holistic care 106, 121-122, 124, 189, 200
homophobia 98, 107, 109
homosexual experience 6
homosexuality 8, 66-67, 174, 196, 211
    and healthcare 105
    bisexuality 66
homosexuals 199, 202
hormonal treatments 101
housewives 116
human character 118
human immunodeficiency virus 87, 175
human rights 198, 202
    rights violations 98
human sexuality 63-64
    and the normality/abnormality debate within psychology 66
humanistic approach 206, 229
hypocrisy 115, 122, 196
hysterical woman 161
hysterisation of women's bodies 161

I

identification of sexual health needs 123
illegal and immoral 21
illness-related 52
images 127, 140, 147, 149, 153
immortality 41
inaccurate advice 83
incest 128, 138, 144, 152
infection pool 212

informal discourses 5, 16
innocent victims 78
instinctual force 160
integrity 105
intellectual functioning 159
Interactionists 14, 16
Intermediate level 230
interpretations of scriptures 104
interventions 160, 218, 227, 228
Iolaus 96
Is childbirth sexual 82
isolation 201
issue of pleasure 169

K

Kinsey 48, 62, 64-65
    reports 12

L

law 40, 103
    and order 173
LBL 30
learning
    about sexuality 116
    difficulty 199
    disabilities 159-160, 176
    disabled 160
legal
    and moral 21
    framework 124
    prescription of normality 167
    right 178
    yet immoral 21
lesbian 95
    custody cases 104
    issues 100
    sex 103
    women 85, 87, 97, 98, 101, 199, 202
Lesbian Information Service 103
life experience 230
lobotomy 100
Local Government Act 102
local population agendas 211
London Lighthouse 101
loss of control 201
LYSIS 103

M

macrosocial issues 12
mainstream religious churches 105
male
    approval 119
    bias 77
    control 221

dominance 77
homosexuals 97
model of sexuality 82
power 6
tyranny 167
world view 164
malfunction
  physical 196
  psychological 196
Malthusian
  couple 161
  fear 162
management of the population 162
management
  policies 175
  support 175
Managing the population: the feeble-minded and sexual perverts 162
marginalisation of sexuality 189
marriage 105
masculine norm 79
masculine-dominated scientific approach 89
masturbating child 161
media 122
  coverage 4
  coverage of sexuality 200
  scandals 151
medical
  interventions 209
  logic 196
  model 76
  model basis 120
  model of childbirth 82
medicalisation v health promotion 214
medication 173, 175
medicine and psychiatry of sexuality 48
meeting sexuality needs 202
men with learning disabilities 165
mental health 173
  and sexuality xv
  problems 173, 175-176, 183
Mental Health Act (1983) 101
Mental Health Foundation 103
mental illness 101
methodology 218
methods of working xiii
microsocial
  aspects 14
  questions 12
middle-class
  culture 33
  values 29
midwives 89

Miller 144, 152
Mims-Swenson Sexual Health Model 226, 228, 229, 231-232
MIND 102
model of nursing 123
monitoring 217
monogamy 7
moral
  arguments 40
  community 25, 26
  decline 129, 131
  respectability 162
  right 178
  state 17, 26
  system 95
  themes 163
mortality and morbidity rate 130-131
motherhood 75, 132-133, 141-142, 156, 163
motivation 63
multidimensional perspective 83
mysterious' force of nature 4
myth of childhood happiness 127, 129, 137, 139
myths 232

N

national differences 31
National Survey of Sexual Attitudes and Lifestyles 221
NATO 102
natural roles 163
nature
  of being 41
  of knowledge 41
NAZ 101
negative
  attitudes 107
  stereotyping 203
negotiation 14
  of care 123
negotion strategies
  protection 33
  selection 33
neurohormone 83
neuroleptics 174
new technologies 55
noble doctor 48
nominalistic psychiatry 48
non-judgmental care 123, 198
non-sexual disabilities 50
normal 49, 72
  sexual behaviour 69
nosology of sexual disorder 52

The nurse's attitudes, beliefs and value systems 198
nurse education 121-122, 204-205, 227, 231
nurse educator 225
nurse's role 202
nurse-patient relationship 105
nursing
    behaviour 203
    curriculum 204
    models 122
    practice 204, 225
    texts 227

O

objective epistemology 43
obsessive sexual ritual 169
Oedipal
    complex 117
    phase 117
Oedipus and Electra
    theories 77
off-street prostitution 27
outcome 221
    measures 219, 221
outlets 13
outline a suitable curriculum model xvi
overt biological signals 79
oxytocin 84

P

PACE 101
paedophiles 10
paid employment 164
paraphilia 68
Parliament of 1982 101
patients' rights 106, 200, 201
patriarchal
    authority 164
    values 164
    heterosexual, nuclear family 163
patriarchy 81, 87
pedagogisation of children's sex 161
peer group play 6
pelvic inflammatory disease 212
penis envy 77
pension schemes 103
people with
    learning disabilities 163, 164, 168-169
    mental health problems 176
perception of risk 215
perfect sex acts 3
personal identity 99

personal liberties 178
personality 192-193, 195
perverse adult 161, 165
phallic primacy 64
phenomenolog 44
philosophers 55
philosophical
    approach 41-42, 55-56
    perspective 40
    puzzle 42
philosophy 40-41, 55
physically disabled 199
physiological 75
    factors 175
    responses 89
Piaget 116
planning of practitioner education 228
Plato 47-48, 96
P-LI-SS-IT model 228
police 16
policies xv, 176
political agenda 225
polyandry 7
polygamy 7
polymorphously perverse 64
Poor Laws 163
postmodernism 44
post-pubescent homosexual sex 65
power 6
power-neutral 6
preconceptions 232
pregnancies 75, 82, 115
prejudices 206, 232
principles of justice 20
privacy 18
The problem of assessment 217
process evaluation 217
process of learning 217
Professional Sexual Role Inventory 204
professional training 175
Project Sigma 30
promiscuity 122, 211
promoting sexual health 219
pronatalist values 164
prostitution 211
psychiatrisation of perverse pleasures 161
psychiatry 61-62, 66, 70-71, 173
psychical hermaphroditism 63
psychoanalysis 44, 64
psychoanalysts 78
psychoanalytic themes 77, 100

psychological 75
    perspectives 76
    disturbance 67
    impairment 199
    tests 100
psychologist 180
psychology 61-62, 66, 70-71
    of personal perception 51
psychosexual
    attraction 13
    functioning 98
psychosocial aspects 81
psychotherapy 67
psychotropic drugs 174, 175, 181
public opinion and public policy 98
public regulation 163
publications 227
pure sciences 8

Q

questions of existence 56

R

randomised control trials 218
Rawls 19
RCTs 218-219
redefining
    abnormality 71
    normality 69
reflective tool 229, 237
regime of truth 9
religion and homosexuality 104
religious dogma 196
reluctant to discuss sexuality xiii
reproduction 163
reproductive health 209
research 175, 227
rights battles 24
rigorous scientific methodology 64
risk 216
    behaviour 216, 218, 221
    reduction 218
role
    differentiation 116
    models 99, 164
    play 99, 182, 230
Roman Empire 96
Roman same-sex relationships 96
Rorschach ink blot tests 100
Royal College of Psychiatrists 102

S

safer sex 17, 177, 182, 210, 214, 216, 220
safety 176

same-sex
    lovers 96
    orientation 97
    relationships 95, 98, 107
    sexual behaviour 97
Sartre 44
schizophrenia 173, 180-182
school education 100
scientific perspective 77
scrupulous ethics 197
segregated groups 160
segregation 123
self- 195
    actualisation 206
    assessment 228
    awareness 226
    belief 189
    concept 119
    confidence 119
    consciousness 119
    designation 49
    empowerment 211
    esteem 118-119, 123
    identity 166
    image 118, 125, 193, 195, 205
    monitoring 198
    referral 212
    respect 193
    worth 195
sensory impaired 199
sensual experience of breast-feeding 84
seroconversion rates 220
set of practices 49
setting targets 218
seven-point continuum 13
sex
    economy 44
    education 124-125, 159
    role behaviour 116
    role stereotypes 116
    therapist 180
sex-obsessed culture 4
sexual
    abnormality 48
    abstinence 85
    abuse 86-87
    actualisation 189
    aggressors 78
    arousal 65
    aspects of childbirth 89
    assault 176
    autonomy 77
    behaviour 202
    boundaries 182

categories 96
citizenship 17, 25
culture 24
decision-making 215
disorders 67
division of labour 116
dysfunctions 68
exploitation 175-176
fix 3
freedom 202
functioning 174
harassment 176
health 24, 40, 49-51, 54, 56, 115, 120-122, 159, 161, 209, 211, 226, 227, 232
    health advice 177
    a mental state 51
    as a physical state 49
    health as a set of practices 47
    health as an instinctual drive 46
    health as societal well-being 53
    health development 226
    health needs 125, 180
    health programme 177
    health promotion 115, 175, 209-210, 225
    health promotion in mental health 176
    health promotion in the context of HIV/AIDS 209
    healthcare 180, 192
    history 180
    hypocrisy 197
    identity 161, 168, 214
    impulses 63
    information 192
    innuendo 5
    knowledge 24
    liberalisation 174
    normality 195-196
    orientation 66
    relationships 177, 183
    risk-taking 215
    role 189
    scripts 215
    side-effects 175
    therapy 65
Sexual Behaviour in Britain Study 221
Sexual citizenship and dimensions of sexual health 24
sexualised therapist-patient relationships 182
sexuality 75, 80, 117, 119, 159, 165, 175, 180, 189, 191, 193, 195, 199-201, 203-206, 209, 212, 225-227, 229, 231-232
    and child care 120
    and nurse education 227
    and nursing care 203
    and the well-being of the individual 192
    belief and value systems 195
    education 225
    in a sociocultural context 61
    in pregnancy 75
    needs 202
    pleasure and identity 166
Sexuality — towards a nursing definition 190
sexually
    abusive behaviour 176
    aggressive 80
    ignorant 127, 133
    transmitted diseases 50, 87, 106, 115, 175, 177, 192, 209-211
SHAKTI 101
short-hand stereotypes 5
side-effects 174
similarities and differences between humans and non-human primates 79
Simone de Beauvoir 44
simplistic sexual models 168
single parenthood 131
slang 5
Snowball sampling 30
social
    cleansing 103
    constraints 121
    construction 11, 56, 89, 161
    construction of masculinity 164
    construction of sexualities 8, 12
    constructionalist 160
    control 159
    disorder 62
    isolation 168
    phenomenon xiv
    prejudices 107
    psychology 205
    roles 163
    structure 54
    support 99
    surveillance 162
    workers 16
    worth 193
socialisation
    of nurses 121
    of procreative behaviours 161
    process 121

constructed 81
society 189, 195-196
Society of Friends or Quakers 105
socio-biology 47
sociological
    perspectives 76
    focus 8
sperm donations 87
spiritual
    dimension 104
    well-being 104
Spock 145-146
Squarcialupi Report 102
staff guidelines 176
standards prevailing in society 23
static labels 96
STD clinics 29
STDs 124, 175, 183, 210, 213, 215
stereotypes 104, 107, 203, 232
stereotypic attitudes 106, 121
stigma 99, 107, 212-213
Stonewall Immigration Group 103
Stonewall Riots 65
student-centred approaches 225
study of sexuality 76
subordination 6
suicide 99
support 210
support teachers 99
surveillance 213
survivors of sexual abuse or rape 85

T

taboo 121, 173, 196, 200, 206
target needs 211
tax inspectors 15
teaching of sexuality 228
teaching techniques 160
techniques of normalisation 162
teenage fathers 137
teenage pregnancy 128, 130-131, 134
telephone help lines 99
Terence Higgins Trust 101, 209
the anti-psychology approach 71
The way forward 122
Theory of
    female sexuality 76
    heredity 162
    Natural Selection 62

therapeutic
    conditions 182
    relationship 177, 180
tolerance 98
traditional views 204
training 176
transcendence 50
Truby King 142
truisms 8
Trust, intimacy and personal autonomy 215

U

understanding cultural diversity 69
unethics 219
US Panel on the Evaluation of AIDS Interventions 220
use of 'cute' children 5

V

value
    judgments 203
    systems 189, 195-196, 198
victimisation 99
victims 3
    of abuse 176
violence 78, 98
virtuous society 197
vulnerability 201

W

Watson 143
welfare services 164, 169
welfare state 162
welfare state support 163
western
    attitudes 105
    pathology 62
    philosophical tradition 39
WHO 222
witches 77
Wolfenden legal watershed 20
Wolfenden Report 17-18, 101
women with learning disabilities 164
working-class 29
Working-class culture 33
workshop activities 230
workshops 228
World Health Organization 101, 198, 202, 210, 217, 227